Praise for *Whole Body Healing*

"*Whole Body Healing* is an inspiring and interactive guide for anyone ready and willing to experience their innate wholeness. Guiding readers through a plethora of diverse practices, Emily is a wise and empathetic lead to follow. Having taken her own healing journey, she shows us all how to go the distance with conviction and love."

—Jennie Lee, author of *Breathing Love* and *True Yoga*

"The information in this book can change our understanding of how our mind, body, and spirit impact our whole-body wellness, and that we can make simple changes for dramatic healings. In this inspiring book, Emily Francis gives us an evolved understanding of the roadblocks that makes us ill, and how we can use this advanced knowledge combined with modern energy healing techniques to heal our body, mind & spirit."

—Marianne Pestana, host of *Moments with Marianne*

"Our bodies are innately brilliant and its wisdom is available if we learn to listen. In *Whole Body Healing*, Emily Francis shows us how weaving the wisdom of the body, the mind and spirit can lead us into our fullest, healthiest, most vibrant lives."

—Dayna Macy, author of *Ravenous*

"*Whole Body Healing* is a road map for readers who wish to get at the root cause of disease and take charge of their health with science-based healing advice. It is a comprehensive and completely useful guide for those widely choosing to positively modulate their health. Emily tells us how to influence the evolution of our bodies and minds toward maximum health and consequent enjoyment of life. A must-read for anyone wanting to live better longer."

—Elisa Lottor, PhD, HMD, author of *The Miracle of Regenerative Medicine*

"Emily Francis presents a well-balanced approach to creating healing miracles for yourself and those you love … She offers both pragmatic and spiritual perspectives on how to create significant improvement, even when doctors say it can't be done. Whatever you are seeking to balance, the answer lies in healing the whole self from the inside out … I wholeheartedly recommend *Whole Body Healing* as an excellent resource and guidebook on your healing path."

—Sarah Shockley, author of *The Pain Companion*

"How does miraculous healing happen? And more importantly, how can we bring healing—spontaneous and otherwise—into our own lives? A tale of tenacity and unwavering belief, this book is a blueprint for healing in the modern world—it takes us beyond traditional and alternative medicine and into the unlimited potentialities of the soul."

—Sara Wiseman, author of *Messages from the Divine*

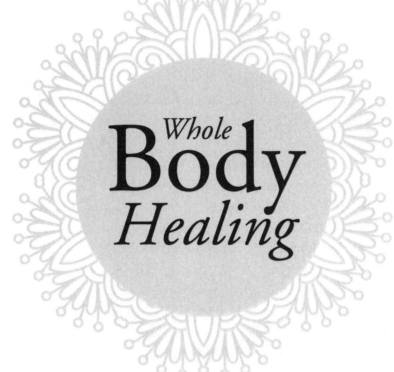

Whole
Body
Healing

About the Author

Emily A. Francis is the host of the weekly internet radio show *All About Healing* on Healthy Life Radio (www.healthylife.net). She is the author of *The Body Heals Itself: How Deeper Awareness of Your Muscles and Their Emotional Connection Can Help You Heal* (Llewellyn, 2017) and coauthor of *Witchy Mama: Magickal Traditions, Motherly Insights & Sacred Knowledge* with Melanie Marquis (Llewellyn, 2016). She is also the author of the book *Stretch Therapy: A Comprehensive Guide to Individual and Assisted Stretching* (Blue River Press, 2012) and is currently under contract for the book *Healing Ourselves Whole* (HCI Publishing, June 2021).

Emily holds a Masters of Science in Physical Education with a concentration in Human Performance and a Bachelor of Science in Exercise Science and Wellness with a minor in nutrition both from Jacksonville State University where she was a collegiate cheerleader. She is a graduate of the Atlanta School of Massage in Clinical and Neuro-muscular therapy. She then went on to graduate through all levels of training at the Dr. Vodder School North America in Manual Lymphatic Drainage and Combined Deconges-tive Therapy (MLD/CDT). She completed level 1 and 2 of Craniosacral Therapy through the Upledger Institute and is a certified Pediatric Therapist through Tina Allen and the Little Kidz Foundation.

Emily completed 300 hours of yoga teacher training in the Sivananda style of yoga (Universal Yoga) under her teacher, Dattattreya, the senior disciple of Swami Vishnude-vananda. She began practicing both yoga and tai chi in the late 1990s and she holds a gold medal in tai chi form from the 2001 US Open, a bronze medal in Push Hands from the same competition, and a silver medal in push hands from the National Taiji Legacy tournament that same year. She is both a Usui and Karuna Ki Reiki Master Level practi-tioner and teacher. You can find Emily at www.emilyafrancisbooks.com.

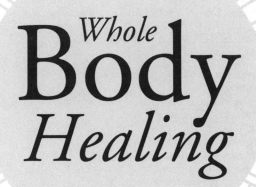

Whole Body Healing

Create Your *Own Path* to
*Physical, Emotional, Energetic
& Spiritual Wellness*

EMILY A. FRANCIS

Llewellyn Publications
Woodbury, Minnesota

First Edition
First Printing, 2020

Cover design by Shannon McKuhen
Figurative illustrations by Mary Ann Zapalac
Somatic Emotion Chart on page 120 by Llewellyn Art Department

Llewellyn is a registered trademark of Llewellyn Worldwide Ltd.

Library of Congress Cataloging-in-Publication Data (Pending)
Names: Francis, Emily A., author.
Title: Whole body healing : create your own path to physical, emotional,
    energetic & spiritual wellness / Emily A. Francis.
Description: First edition. | Woodbury, Minnesota : Llewellyn Publications,
    2020. | Includes bibliographical references and index. | Summary:
    "Summary: For people interested in alternative health, shows a more
    science-related approach to mind-body-spirit healing as part of an
    integrated whole"-- Provided by publisher.
Identifiers: LCCN 2019059145 (print) | LCCN 2019059146 (ebook) | ISBN
    9780738762180 (paperback) | ISBN 9780738762524 (ebook)
Subjects: LCSH: Alternative medicine. | Mind and body.
Classification: LCC R733 .F782 2020 (print) | LCC R733 (ebook) | DDC
    610--dc23
LC record available at https://lccn.loc.gov/2019059145
LC ebook record available at https://lccn.loc.gov/2019059146

Llewellyn Publications
A Division of Llewellyn Worldwide Ltd.
2143 Wooddale Drive
Woodbury, MN 55125-2989
www.llewellyn.com

Printed in the United States of America

Other Books by Emily A. Francis

The Body Heals Itself: How Deeper Awareness of Your Muscles and Their Emotional Connection Can Help You Heal (Llewellyn, 2017)

Witchy Mama: Magickal Traditions, Motherly Insights & Sacred Knowledge with Melanie Marquis (Llewellyn, 2016)

Stretch Therapy: A Comprehensive Guide to Individual and Assisted Stretching (Blue River Press, 2012)

Forthcoming Books by Emily A. Francis

Healing Ourselves Whole (HCI Publishing, June 2021)

Dedication

I dedicate this book to each and every one of you.
Thank you for joining this journey with me.
Remember Always…

You Are Capable
You Are Fierce
You Are Powerful
You Are Mighty
Your Intuition Is on Point
You Can Rock Any Challenge That Comes Your Way
You Deserve to Live a Happy and Healthy Life
Don't
Ever
Stop

Acknowledgments

Thank you God, my Angels, and Guides.

Thank you: Scott, Hannah, Ava, and the rest of my family for being everything I love most in this world.

Thank you to everyone at the Upledger Institute for your incredible support of my work. Forever I will hold dear what you have given to our family.

To my team at Llewellyn: Having people such as yourselves is invaluable in bringing this book into the world. Thank you: Angela Wix and Kat Sanborn.

Thank you: Paul Levine, literary agent.

Thank you for the endorsements and support of this work: Amy B. Scher, Sara Wiseman, Jennie Lee, Dayna Macy, Elisa Lottor, Sarah Shockley, and Marianne Pestana.

Sincere gratitude for your contributions and insight: Dr. Rachel Jack, Jessica Silva, Kristina Duffy, and Lindy Pals.

And an incredible thank you to those who joined me for a weekend in the mountains to help me brainstorm as well as offer incredible knowledge and insights for the creation of this work. I purposely chose the best of the best to help me create a full and detailed offering of healing practices through each of you. That weekend will mean more to me than I can possibly express. I will only list by name and not credentials because there are too many following each of your names to share! Thank you: Tom Dill, Tami Goldstein, David Mitchell, Carola Kauffhold, Stephen Watson, Heather Hale, Ashli Callaway, Eden Callaway. Thank you: Bonnie Cole for your gift of handmade mala beads that helped make that weekend so very special. Lastly, a special thank you and love to the one we've lost between that weekend and the publication of this book, Pamela Bellamy. The world will never look quite the same without you in it. I pray you are dancing in the light joyfully on the other side.

Contents

Practices

Chapter 7

Chapter 8

Chapter 9

Chapter 10

Chapter 11

Chapter 14

Foreword

*Y*ou have the ability to heal. I know this to be true. But I also know this isn't always easy to hear. When people used to offer me the same idea, especially during my worst moments of illness, I wanted so badly to believe it. But I was also scared to entertain its truth because a small voice inside me wondered, *What if I can't do it? What if healing is for everyone else, but not me?*

In 2010, after suffering with chronic, debilitating Lyme disease for almost a decade, I had an epiphany: if I wanted to truly heal, I was going to have to go beyond chasing a physical cure. I had literally traveled around the world seeking various treatments—from Los Angeles to Chicago and even to India. In addition to Lyme disease, I had dozens of other conditions: autoimmune thyroid, brain lesions, neuropathy, arthritis, and more. I was only in my twenties, but my body was falling apart. It was clear to me that my current methods of trying to gain my life and health back were not working. The alternative to my failed attempts at letting others heal me was a truth I could not ignore: I was going to have to, somehow, heal myself. The only problem was that I had no idea *how*. Overwhelmed by physical symptoms and the emotional challenges that come along with chronic illness, I sometimes lacked the confidence to believe I could even get through the day, let alone fix my broken body.

What I discovered is that it can be done; perhaps not always with ease and grace, but even so. What you need is a path. And this rare gem of a book, *Whole Body Healing,* is here to offer you exactly that. But what is unique about this book is that it does not just provide you *the* path. It gives you the training you need to discover *your* own path to become your own greatest healer.

Whole Body Healing will help you address *every* aspect of yourself: physical, energetic, emotional, and spiritual. But it continues where most books leave off by showing you how to integrate all you have learned into one seamless approach.

I wish I'd had Emily and this book during my own healing journey. When you are lost, sick, and scared, everything feels like too much. But here, Emily takes what can feel impossible and makes it doable. She feels like the best friend, the mother, and the soul sister that everyone longs for. In the healing space Emily provides, there is no room for "no." Where some see dead ends, Emily sees only more doors. And she'll stand by them right with you.

After healing myself permanently and completely using a self-created mind-body approach, I can confirm wholeheartedly what Emily shares in her work: there is no single prescription for healing.

Emily teaches you, based on your own individuality, to align with the methods and approaches that are best for *you*. She gives you the tools, techniques, and confidence to integrate the best that all medicines have to offer: natural, allopathic, and your own sacred intuition.

In a world where it's easy to lose touch with the rhythms and needs of our own bodies, Emily guides you back to the wisdom we all possess inside. And once you have that, you have everything.

There may be times along the way when things feel scary or hard. But I know that with Emily by your side, you can do this.

Now, go claim your whole body health. You deserve it. And, it's been waiting for you all along.

Amy B. Scher
Author of *How to Heal Yourself When No One
Else Can* (Llewellyn Worldwide, 2016), *This Is
How I Save My Life* (Simon & Schuster, 2018),
and other books on human-ing and healing.

Introduction

You are powerful beyond your imagination. You are highly capable of making extraordinary shifts in your life. Your body's ability to heal is so much greater than anyone has ever permitted you to believe. Set the intention now that you have the power within yourself to heal, grow, recover, discover, create, and expand through every level of your being. I believe in you.

I believe in miracles and miracle healing. I believe that when we tap into our source of Divine guidance, as well as learn to truly gather solid information from which to make each decision, our whole world can balance out in ways we may not have experienced before. I personally have experienced miracle healings more than once in my life. First, with my own long and very hard-earned recovery from severe anxiety and panic. Second, with the recovery of my daughter out of her autism spectrum diagnosis.

When I refer to miracle healing, please understand that this in no way implies that it was quick. We did not wake up healed. That is defined as *spontaneous healing*. I believe in that too, but that has not been my personal experience in my journey. We did not get struck by a healing lightning bolt that changed everything in our bodies. We were a vital part of our miracle making. The reason I think of my own personal recovery as miraculous is because I truly experience life now the way that I did before anxiety ever took it over. There were many years where I never thought that was possible. Once my mind and body could remember what it was like without debilitating fear, it locked into all body systems to provide lasting effects. I worked harder than I could possibly explain for my recovery.

Working for my daughter's recovery was a much clearer process. I was so much more determined to find the right combination for her healing, and this time I knew how to go about it from the start. It felt as if my instincts kicked in right at the onset. I put my head down and got to work to find exactly the right healing combination for her. Maybe I went through my own years of healing and researching so that when I had my daughter and her diagnosis came up, I would have all the tools in place to help her reach her full healing potential in a fairly direct line of passage.

With regard to recovering my child, we were led down exactly the right paths to help her brain reorganize itself and heal from the inside out. It was nothing short of blissful insanity what we witnessed for her with each right door we opened. Even though the span was just two years, the places we went for treatment and for diagnosis felt like we packed twenty years of testing and procedures into it. It was a series of nonstop efforts and searches for who could help us. I knew in my heart that I could help her recover. I knew already being in the healing field, I had a heck of a head start. I had no idea how that process would look. I had to approach our healing with blind faith that, somehow, we would find our way.

What brought it all together, especially in my quest for my child's healing, was learning how to communicate with Spirit by asking to be led to each next best step. There were usually responses to big prayer requests while laying hands on my child in the middle of the night, or through tears of aggravation and complete despair of what to do next. None of this was pretty, but the results were amazing. The journey was not nearly as tidy as it is being laid out here. Spirit led the way, and I listened. That is my best explanation for our process. It's also what I intend to teach you through this book. The primary goal is to follow the guidance from deep within and not get lost in the sea of voices that comes with letting too many people in where deep healing is concerned.

An Experience in Healing

Healing is messy and requires a vicious tenacity to keep attempting to go layer after layer deeper into the void of oneself. Do not mistake my miracle explanations for anything less than disciplined and faithful beliefs that there had to be something more to our lives than what we were experiencing. With that notion in mind, we never gave up. Watching my child come to life in high definition was the greatest gift of my life. If I had ever questioned the power of miracles, the boundless opportunities that the body has to heal itself *if given the right tools,* I had no doubts of it now.

My daughter's healing occurred through the process of writing my most recent book *The Body Heals Itself: How Deeper Awareness of Your Muscles and Their Emotional Connection Can Help You Heal.* I was led to all the right places to interview for my book, though its focus was emotional muscle memory, not autism or anything similar. Through the process of writing, I gained access into more healing modalities than I had ever previously known. What I found in that process changed our lives forever. We had been blessed with the greatest miracle of our lives, and my book about healing had not even been released!

What the path of writing that book brought to us was having the same developmental pediatrician who diagnosed my child say to me that she no longer met the criteria for an ASD diagnosis! She looked me straight in the eye and said, "This rarely to never happens. You need to claim your miracle and know that everything you're doing is working."

We had her diagnosed through three separate avenues, all resulting in the same ASD mild/moderate with speech apraxia diagnosis. We stuck with our developmental pediatrician beyond the diagnostic practitioners because of the three, she was the one who sent us to the most testing and to other specialists for confirmation. She was the one we most trusted for an unbiased analysis. Therefore, we also returned to her for reevaluations. We also had a second evaluation done through the school system; against their original beliefs, they too agreed with the developmental pediatrician that our daughter does not display any level of autism spectrum disorders.

Strangely, each time I share our story of amazing healing, the people's responses either jump to (1) we were misdiagnosed from the start or (2) we *grew out* of the diagnosis. I call BS on both of those excuses (plus my child was five years old, not twenty-five). Other people say that once someone is on the spectrum, they can never get off. I reply: "Says who?" Who determined this to be a truth that everyone just accepts? I'm keeping our miracle because that is exactly what it is. Never second-guess the gifts the Universe provides, and always believe that you deserve miracle healing. Body healing is entirely possible when you treat the body in full.

What You Will Learn

I share this part of our story to say that through the process of writing my own book and through the process of recovering both myself and my child from different issues, I have done tremendous research into opportunities to heal that lie beyond any standard proto-col. This is the reason why I have chosen to offer this book. I have done the research for you. I will teach you how to get still and learn to tap into your higher wisdom so you can avoid wasting precious healing time listening to too many voices and get moving on your best path to wholeness. I wrote this book in the hopes that when something feels off, you will have enough information to be provided a moment to pause. In this pause, we can discern which aspect of the body we need to focus on and possibly who to go to for help.

It doesn't matter what the diagnosis may be. Healing is available to everyone to improve their quality of life *if* you are willing to go there. In no way does healing guarantee some kind of effect on the length of your life. I can offer you enough tools to figure out for yourself where to go with the foundation of taking each right next step. I will help you not get too ahead of yourself and honor Divine timing for true and lasting healing. When you make the commitment to cut through all the muck in your life for healing, it can be an isolating process. True healing can get messy and requires all of your attention. Had I put myself out there to all my friends and social media for what we were going through, I knew I could get lost in a sea of voices that were not my own. Those voices can be such a distraction that you end up doing circles and never get anywhere in your healing. It is a dangerous cycle to enter, allowing too many voices to guide your way, and it is not my intention with this book. My attempt is to provide the research, teach you how to do your own research, and above all to tap into your own inner wisdom so that you can make choices based on research and instinct in combination.

You do not need to be sick to read this book. This book is not for the sick, nor is it a guide to conquer illness. Instead, it's an offering into any aspect of healing that you might be needing in your life. It will allow you to see your body in full and provide a deeper understanding of what we need to know to make lasting and sustainable changes in order for our greatest good and highest joys to be carried out in this life. It is a blueprint offering for multilevel healing within our bodies and how it operates in this world. Wherever you are today, in this moment, and wherever you want to be, I hope this book will provide the guidance you are seeking in order to help yourself heal from within.

There are a few things to remember:

1. *Nothing in the body operates independently.* Not one part of our body operates alone. When looking at our bodies, we want to approach any level of healing as

all-inclusive. We have to look at the whole body and all its glorious layers and attend to every aspect of the whole.

2. *True and authentic healing comes from within.* No one else can do any of it for you, but they can certainly help. In the end, it is from inside yourself that true and lasting healing can be obtained.

The road to wholeness is different for every person; there is no single prescription for everyone. The lack of knowledge for what is possible concerns me the most. We all need to know that incredible healing opportunities and miracles are all around the world. What you are searching for might not be a mainstream treatment opportunity where you live. But it is a practice from somewhere, and the people who train in those practices don't all live where they trained. You might find that what you are looking for is a block away from where you are, but you just may not know it exists until you start this process. My role here is to offer you the widest amount of research so that you can find what your next right step is, whatever will put you on the path for you or your loved one's healing.

In order to find your specific combination into healing, you must be willing to take off any blinders and search far and wide for the possibilities. Limited vision serves as nothing but a roadblock. If to this point you have not believed in magic … well, take those blinders off, put on a pair of rainbow-colored glasses, and take a good look around you. We live on a ball that circles around a star which happens to be another ball of constant fire and energy—that is magic. Magic, miracles, and opportunities abound when we open up to the endless possibilities that are waiting for us.

Addressing Layers of the Whole Body for Healing

We must be willing to address the entire body in order to have lasting and sustainable results. We have to look at the body from the *physical* dimension and see doctors, therapists, and healers who understand the body's physical aspect.

We also need to understand our *emotional* bodies and how they play a part in our balance and healing. Stuck or displaced emotions can create more health issues than we are generally aware of. The magnitude that our emotions play on our health is enormous. We must be willing to do the work for our emotional body to be able to find the best combination of healing therapies and therapists. Generally, we will not go to the same people for emotional healing we saw for physical relief or testing.

The *energetic* body is something close to the emotional body, but they are not the same. Therefore, you must know how to work with your energy body, the layer where the miracles live. This subtle part of the body is the power player in our ability to heal. We must know how to understand and work with our energy body, as well as activate and balance this aspect.

Last but certainly not least is the *spiritual* component necessary for deep healing. This will bring to you a new field of beings to help you to become conscious of your spirit body and how to use it to manifest deep balance and health. We will gather our "spirit team" (as I refer to them). Cultivating a spiritual practice is a vital piece of this journey to whole body healing. When all of these various aspects of your body are put into motion with the same intention to heal, miracles come to life.

As we review these layers that make up the whole body, I not only offer introductions into therapies for the body, mind, emotions, energy, and spirit, but also guide you on how to discern which therapist to choose in each related field.

Things won't always be easy, nor will your process always remain neat and clear. I have great faith in your ability to heal. I want you to believe in your ability to heal too. Finally, the key to this whole process is getting to the point where you are able to give yourself permission to heal. Never underestimate the role this part plays. It's the factor that will determine if any of the other offerings will work. It's not just the icing, it's the foundation to the process.

Being able to come back to life and live out loud is a gift that each and every person should have the opportunity to achieve. Sometimes it's learning how to get out of our own way and change our inner dialogue and belief systems. Other times it's finding the right people to treat you and help your body remember how to heal itself. It's finding what the real problems are and from where in your body they are issuing. Above all, the combination for lasting and authentic healing is in addressing every part of the whole, treating all aspects of your health and body. In so doing, it means that there is never just one person you need to go to for your healing. It's finding the right combination to treat every aspect of your body so that you can fully heal and transform your life. It's treating your physical, emotional, and energy bodies as well as learning to work with Divine wisdom to help guide you to all the right people and inspire decisions. In the end, it comes down to gathering proper information and then going with your gut. In this book we will dive into each aspect of the body and learn to tap into our inner voice for guidance.

I believe in your healing. I believe everything is possible. Don't back down until you get all the answers and information that you need. If it's meant to be yours, you still must do the work in order to bring it to life. Hold on tight to your dreams and your convictions to shift and heal. Do what you need to in order to live your very best life. I have faith in you.

Your shift begins here.

Part I

Whole Body Integration

You are magnificent and worthy of whole body healing. Your life is waiting for you to claim it and live it wide open. You can do anything. You are magic. You deserve all the grand offerings that this life can offer. Go get it, warrior! You got this.

Chapter 1

Setting Yourself Up
for Healing

You are already whole. Your body is full of magic and wisdom. I will repeat that sentiment throughout this book to emphasize it, because it's the absolute truth. First acknowledge that nothing is missing, even if sometimes you feel like you aren't able to find it. Everyone in the world finds themselves out of sync with their lives at times, whether within their physical bodies, their emotions, their spiritual practice, or their energy in general. Learning how to discern where an imbalance originates and then finding the path to helping the whole ripple effect rebalance is this book's primary purpose. Many times, we run ourselves in circles trying to figure out how to heal ourselves but simply haven't learned that each aspect of the body requires a totally different approach. Although sometimes cleverly hidden, within each of us is a blueprint that can unlock the greatest healing potential known to humankind. It's all right here within us just waiting to be discovered.

The single most important offering that I could share through this book is the sincere hope and trust in our healing. There is not enough of that in this world. Also, in this book you will be offered the maps to help you navigate your way through each aspect of your body in order to effectively understand and nourish it more fully. You do not need to be sick in any form to read this book and improve your overall well-being. We are all on a journey to living our best lives through the vessel with which we have been blessed to navigate life.

Often when something arises, we don't know where to begin our journey to help ourselves feel whole and healthy. Hopefully this book will offer you a deeper insight into what might be out of balance and from where that issue is signaling. From there, we will learn how to take our best approach to shift and elevate for the imbalances to correct. For example, if we are feeling anxious or depressed, it's not something that our general practitioner can treat as effectively as someone who is trained to work with our emotions, such as a cognitive therapist, psychologist, psychiatrist, or psychotherapist. If it's something out of balance with our energy, the treatment is different, and would require the help of a specialist such as an acupuncturist, Ayurvedic practitioner, yoga teacher, or learning disciplines such as meditation, yoga, tai chi, qi gong, dance, or other spiritually driven movement practices to balance the energy system. If the issue is something physical, we will learn to navigate our way through in order to find a proper diagnosis from the correct specialist. This also entails the body treatments such as chiropractic, massage therapy, herbal remedies, and any other treatment for the physical aspect of the self. Finally, cultivating a spiritual practice is vital to this process for us to learn to follow the guidance and wisdom that go beyond human interpretation.

Taking care of yourself is crucial, be it a physical practice such as a detox or a body treatment, an emotional wellness treatment such as therapy, seeing someone to help balance your energy, going to a meditation center, or even simply going to church to help meet your spiritual needs. There are a lot of little additions you can incorporate into your self-care practice that will make a big difference, and they don't have to break the bank. We must learn to put ourselves up at the top of our priority list so that we can be fully able to give love to others in our lives.

There is a formula for healing and shifting your life that applies to every single person on earth. That formula is to treat every aspect of the whole in order to affect real change within oneself. We may choose different avenues within this context for healing our whole selves. There is an infinite amount of options under each of the aspects to choose from. Each person will be drawn to various opportunities from each aspect. It comes down to following the formula of treating the whole person and everything that this encompasses. That is how we become wholly healed. Know that miraculous and amazing things are entirely possible for us all. That said, there must be a willingness to do the work. Even if something is meant to be yours, you still have to do the work to bring it to life. Healing isn't something that happens to you—it's something that happens *with* you.

Treating the Memory Systems of the Body

We are born with an intelligence that each part of the body knows what it feels like to work at its healthiest and optimal levels, and that knowledge never goes away—it's in the body somewhere, so it's up to us to help it remember when life happens and parts of it forgets. I must preface this by saying that while not every health issue can be restored once it has come all the way up into the level of diagnosis, feeding into the body memory can significantly affect the quality from which it operates. I believe there are several different memory systems within the body, and feeding them good habits can help them to remember what it was like to work at their best levels. Our minds contain memory. Our muscles and other soft tissues of the body contain memory. We are familiar with the idea of cellular memory as well. Different actions lead to feeding different memory systems both independently and together. Getting in tune and balancing the emotions helps to both stimulate and regulate all the memory systems, but in different ways. They all work off each other. To feed a memory system is not a one-step rule that affects everything in the same manner. To change the body's memory system of how it feels when off balance verses how it feels when healthy requires constant effort for a prolonged duration of time. It needs to be long enough that each individual part of the whole-body system is able to remember the true nature of its ability to function well. Seeing is believing is one thing, but internally feeling and remembering is something much deeper. Each aspect of the whole must be fed the proper nourishment for the length each part requires to change the patterns within. Nourishment meaning food, thought patterns, choices, exercise, stress control, even medicine when necessary. Nothing in the body operates independently, but it is still important to relate to the little parts as well as the whole. Be willing to lock a higher form of living into your memory systems. Your body will remember and help hold yourself accountable to continuing to live from that space.

Defining Your Intentions

Take time to answer the questions that follow, and refer back to your answers later on as you continue on your healing journey. These questions are about your intentions, which you may occasionally forget as time goes on, or they could change as situations arise.

⌘ Practice: Questions to Ask Yourself

The first step in beginning the healing path is to define your intentions for your health, for your life, and for the process you are about to create. There are three major questions you must be willing to answer in order to become clear on where you really want to be in your life. I constantly use them to evaluate what I'm really trying to achieve. The questions are:

1. *Who am I?* This means deep inquiry into who you really are, what you are about, and what you stand for. What is really important to you in your personal life, professional life, and in your healing? What are you doing with your time on earth? Do you have a peaceful attitude toward how you are spending your time regarding your personal purpose? Is your health helping to propel you or is it currently a stumbling block?
2. *What do I want?* This one is huge. What are the outcomes that you really want to see happen in your life? The number one intention for the purpose of this book with this question is your body and your health. Are you currently doing what's necessary to live a happy and healthy life? Are your habits lending themselves to your greatest good and highest joy and ultimate healing? If not, you need to be willing to ask and answer the question of what it is you truly want. Be very specific when you answer this question. After you've asked this for your health, use this to navigate every aspect of your life: health, career, relationships, finances, and so on.
3. *What am I willing to do to get it?* This is biggest question and predictor of all, the game changer to the previous two questions. There was a time when I thought about opening a women's center for pre- and post-natal massage therapy as well as post-breast or post-ovarian cancer. I already had most of the training to work with it, so it seemed like an obvious next step. I thought I could create a full-scale women's healing facility based in clinical, hands-on therapy. I thought I could even have a kid's corner to provide childcare while the women were being treated. It all sounded so dreamy and wonderful, but once I started reading the massage business manuals and everything that went into writing the business plan itself, I realized that I was not willing to do the work required to make my dream a reality. In fact, I realized

that I didn't want to be working all day long in any practice at all! When it came to finishing my graduate degree or writing my books, I was willing to do all the things required to make it happen. That is why this is the big defining question. You must always follow up when you are defining your dreams and goals and ask *what am I willing to do to get it?* Lots of people talk about the books they want to write. Few ever complete a book and get it off to print, self-published or otherwise. It takes so much continued effort to continue showing up and work on the same idea over and over again. If it really is what you want, then it becomes something you *have* to do, not just something you *want* to do. When it comes to your health and healing, you may be tasked with having to completely alter your diet, exercise, sleep, and therapies in order to achieve what you truly want the outcome to be. In other words, the answer to *what are you willing to do to get it* will make or break this process. You need to be brutally honest about what you are willing and not willing to do in order to reach the intended results. This question isn't intended to induce guilt; the point is not to make you feel bad if what you are willing to do doesn't measure up to the *What do you want?* question. It means that if you are not willing to do exactly what is required in order to get what you want, then what you want may not be entirely accurate. Reevaluate again and again. This is a personal process, one that no one has any business being a part of answering but you. Be honest with yourself and revisit this practice often.

You do know your answers, even though you might have to listen deeply to the still, small voice within to retrieve them. You need to constantly reevaluate those answers. Be sure to get to quiet spaces as often as you can to hear them. I make every decision in my life based on what feels good to my gut/soul and trust my instincts completely. Though it took years to get to that level, it's such an empowered place to be, and I want it for you too. You are strong and capable, and listening to your own wisdom and your feelings will always guide you well. Trust what comes through to you. Work hard to minimize second-guessing or asking other people to make decisions for you. That puts you in a state of imbalance and uncertainty. No one knows better than you what feels best to you. Pay attention to those feelings and thoughts that come through to you. Continue to check in with yourself often to be sure you are clear with your goals and that they haven't changed. Always be true to yourself. Above all things, trust your gut on every decision you make.

If you want to make big changes, keep those intentions close to the chest. Don't share them until they are fully realized or are at least in action. While you are creating and healing, keep the energy tight and locked so that the intention can carry where it needs to go. It needs to bloom. Some people love to put everything out on social media to help keep them honest; if that's how you work, by all means work within those parameters. We shouldn't block things that help gain momentum in our goals. However, it's often the case that sharing intentions with others has the unintended effect of taking the air out of our creative tires. Try to keep your energy and the shifting patterns occurring right now close to your chest. Don't be too quick to share with other people what you are learning and what you are trying to create. Try not to make too many sentences starting with: "I really want to _____," or "I am starting a new project/book/class." Instead, just do them and put them into practice before ever announcing it. Be sure you are going to follow it through before you spread the energy too thin and it all falls apart. Learning to become your own champion minimizes the need to seek approval through others. Talking about it is simply talking. Put things into motion and make the shift from being a dreamer to a doer. The Universe wants to see your actions and not your words. Words such as *intention* have meaning and power, but *actions* lead to change. Make manifesting the new big thing in your life and trust in your process as you turn it into reality.

Giving Yourself Permission to Heal

The greatest hurdles we must overcome are allowing ourselves to heal and believing that we deserve to be happy and free from pain, shame, guilt, sorrow, or anything else we've been carrying around. Giving yourself permission to heal is something that no one can do for you. It is the most vital part of this process. When it comes to situations such as chronic pain or autoimmune illness, there is no single remedy that can remove everything you've been dealing with. I'm not saying we can ever reverse the situation. I am saying that we can make it a whole lot more livable when we change our relationship with it.

Positive behaviors and beliefs will build more of the same. The same goes for the converse. You must decide which way you want to go. Then you have to get on the same team with all the voices in your head. Every cell and fiber of your being must all be in agreement for lasting changes to occur. Start at the space where you give your full body permission to heal and trust that the process will lead you there. You deserve to feel healthy, and free from pain, shame, guilt or grief. Happiness, joy, bliss, centeredness, and empowerment await you on the other side of your struggle.

⌘ Practice: 3-D Vision Board

In order to get on the same team with the big three questions and answers, there are some practices that you can do to help you gain clarity within yourself for each decision. We all know by now that a vision board can be very helpful in honing in on what we really want in our life. A 3-D vision board can make it even more powerful. For the purpose of this practice, we don't want to make a big full poster board-sized vision board; we want to keep it exactly to only one subject and theme. In order to give ourselves permission to heal and move forward into our best life, we must have all of our thoughts and intentions saying and believing exactly the same things. Take it down into simple mantras of affirmation and then bring it to life on a small size 3-D vision board. This paper should be about the size of an 8 x 11 sheet of paper or something similar. Begin first by the layer that covers the entire paper or board. This is basically the background that will support your manifesting of healing this specific issue. It could be the ocean, grass, beaches, mountains—something that covers the whole bottom and gives you a sense of peace and well-being.

Next, put a photo of you at your healthiest somewhere in this board. Some might want it in the center, others might want it someplace else. Just be sure that you are in there and it inspires you. Don't pull people from any magazines; it's not about models or material things or anyone other than *you* and your sacred intention to heal and shift. Many people I know hang on to a special photo that makes them smile when they look at it, as it makes them feel so proud and happy to see this particular time in their life. It's not about losing weight and looking like you did when you were younger, but it *can* be about how you felt at any time in your life before health challenges, relationship heartaches, or big losses had entered your life.

Next, surround your picture with all the things that it would take to get you to where you want to be. If you need life-changing surgery, choose pictures of the hospital and doctors (pull them off the web or search in medical journals) and the things you will need in order to make this a reality. If it's not something medical, pick the photos that you will need to surround yourself as you go along this new path of elevation. What they look like is entirely up to you. Without your conscious choice, the three layers are exactly *who are you*—beach, ocean, grass, mountains—it's a secret place that helps you become peaceful.

Next, the photo of you answers the question *what do you want?* You are now looking at it or being reminded of what you want or how you want to feel. Finally, surrounding yourself with everything that it would take to get you there is the *what are you willing to do to get it* piece. Make them into pictures. Put them on top of each other. Make it a vivid 3-D board. Bring it to life.

This exercise will get on the same team within our thoughts. Every part of the process of creating this vision board is a repetition of words within yourself of exactly what you intend to create. Don't waste any more valuable time trying to muster up the courage to make your changes—do it now. You have everything it takes to make it happen.

Chapter 2
The Five Pillars for Whole Body Wellness

There are five pillars to optimal wellness. If we integrate each of these five avenues for healing, we will find that our approach to whole body wellness will cover every layer specifically covered in the following sections.

Outline for Optimal Wellness

I must preface the next five sections, of diet, sleep, stress control, attitude/mindset, and exercise/movement, with the caveat that while I know a lot about each of these, I do not necessarily have each subject completely mastered. Some of these areas have been a real struggle for me throughout different stages of my life. I am a messy, honest example of what these things look like: I know what to do and how to do it, but I don't put everything I know into practice consistently in my daily life. This is an important piece of honesty to offer. I am not a perfect example of anything I am about to offer, nor would I expect myself to be. Neither do I expect *you* to demand this of yourself. Overachievers fall hard when they don't succeed. In this case, it's about working with these pillars of wellness to achieve a level of balance that can help us achieve a better quality of life.

1. Food and Diet

The first pillar for optimum wellness centers on our diet. Food can be a medicine, a poison, or simply sustenance. Choosing a well-balanced diet filled with leafy greens and other brightly colored vegetables are a staple for good nutrition. Lowering the amounts of

saturated fats, sugars, and processed foods will help you on a healthy path. Organic produce and meats (should you choose to eat meat at all) are always best.

Our attachment to a food pattern is the most important item and its intention to help
us heal. We rely on certain foods not because our body craves them or even because we
like them, but because we have an emotional attachment to the way certain foods make us
feel. Breaking those connections will free your emotional body and your relationship with
food better than any diet ever could. I've been through my fair share of being told what
to eat, when to eat, and how much to weigh. I was a college cheerleader, so I remember
weekly weigh-ins in front of everyone—believe me, I've been through the negative aspects
of worrying about weight. I don't think I could ever become someone who would tell
anyone what they should or should not eat. Many of our collective issues with food do
not come from within ourselves—they come from hurtful statements along the way that
embed into our minds. Those statements then get airtime, as our personal audio reel takes
over and constantly plays it in our head.

When it comes to diet, I want each of us to step away for just a minute and think
about the way we eat, not just what we eat. When you feel overly stressed, depressed, or
bored, do you turn to the cabinets and fridge and start grazing? I sure do. We've heard
the term "emotional eating" and may shrug it off (or it may mean something to you). I
don't want anyone to give up food or use food as a source of punishment to themselves.
I want us all to have a healthy relationship with food. Let's be realistic and say that diet is a
serious issue with many people. The emotional attachment to it is an extremely important
piece to consider as we navigate through our healing.

It is important to note that a large percentage of men and women who are obese were
victims of sexual, verbal, or physical abuse at some point in their lives. The research and
documentation on suffering from childhood sexual trauma and adulthood obesity are far
and wide; some even refer to it as a second assault.[1] As well, an extremely high percent of
women who have issues with eating disorders also end up receiving a bipolar diagnosis at
some point in their lives, though it is unclear which was diagnosed first or if the order of
diagnoses matters. The point is that almost all issues with food stem from an emotional
pattern that was set early in our lives due to something potentially traumatic. "Adolescent

1. Olga Khazan, "The Second Assault" *The Atlantic* (December 15, 2015). https://www.theatlantic.com/health/
archive/2015/12/sexual-abuse-victims-obesity/420186/.

girls who experience physical and sexual dating violence show a relatively high rate of abnormal weight control behaviors that include laxative use and/or vomiting."[2] It could be as simple as something someone says to you that instantly changes the way you view yourself and your body. Many people use excess food to avoid issues of trauma. They opt to become more invisible to the world. This is generally an unconscious decision put into motion. It's important that we bring this issue out into the light. There is so much to be uncovered when it comes to our food choices in correlation to our emotional behaviors. It's not our stomach that is the problem, it's our thoughts. It's our approach. It's our willingness to be proactive and set ourselves up each day for better decision-making skills when it comes to our food choices.

Tips for Who to Look For

I want to take a moment to offer therapies or practices that might be helpful as you navigate your way through this avenue. If you have issues around not eating, binge eating, or feeling guilty when you do eat, then a psychologist, psychotherapist, or psychiatrist might be a good fit for understanding your attachments to food. My personal preferred therapy with issues centering on food and diet is hypnotherapy. Generally, a hypnotherapist has training in psychology, or at least they would be the ones I would seek. They can help you identify the causes and the patterns in which you eat. They can also implement changes within your subconscious mind to help you create a healthier pattern for yourself. The hypnotherapy approach is incredibly powerful, and I highly recommend it.

If you are looking for help with a specific diet to help aid in healing, a nutritionist or dietician would be the way to go. Someone undergoing chemotherapy treatment or who has a compromised immune system is often prescribed what is referred to as a neutropenic diet. This means that they shouldn't eat anything that has not been fully cooked due to the bacteria that might be on the food. This is helpful as a parameter of what not to eat. But what about what you *should* eat? This is where these diet specialists play a crucial role in helping you create the right healing diet for you. If you are facing a health challenge or a health crisis, a dietician or nutritionist with training in your exact issue is highly beneficial to your healing and recovery. You want to find someone who knows all the ins and outs

---

2. Willam D. McArdle, Frank I. Katch, and Victor L. Katch, *Sports and Exercise Nutrition*. Lippincot Williams & Wilkins Fourth Edition (2014), 517.

of your condition to prescribe the diet that can help you recover. Food is medicine, if you allow it be. This can be the game changer in any recovery.

Nutritionists as well as dieticians both evaluate the health of their clients to determine the best foods to eat. Both are considered experts on foods, but the difference is in the level of education, training, and testing. A registered dietician (RD) is registered with the commission on dietetic registration. A nutritionist is a profession that is not as regulated and therefore someone with food training, but not a formal school education, can fall under the scope of being a nutritionist. An RD requires a minimum of a four-year degree of training from an accredited university. Sometimes people prefer a nutritionist to an RD simply because that particular person is better trained to plan a diet that fits their needs. If you find a nutritionist who also has the RD behind their name, even better: they have the hours and credentialed set of training as well as specialized training into the specific avenue of diet you might be looking for (these are referred to as RDNs). If you want to go to someone who really knows their stuff, find someone who went on to specialize in their training beyond the core fundamentals. Any nutritionist, dietician, or health coach can do this. They must do some sort of study beyond their original school in order to truly be of service to specific individual nutrition plans. Above all, it is important to find someone who knows everything there is to know within the one specific practice you are looking for if you want to make a real change.

I recently interviewed author Dayna Macy, author of the book *Ravenous*, on my radio show. She used a spiritual approach to change the way she used food in her life. She said she doesn't believe in going *on* a diet because that would imply that at some point you will also be going *off* that diet. Instead, she opted to develop a healthy relationship with her food. She didn't take anything away, only served herself smaller portions. She practiced asking herself questions like "is this really what my body wants?" She also offered some amazing, profound insight: a yoga teacher once told her that when a body is out of balance, it craves the things that will continue to keep it out of balance. A body that is in balance will continue to crave things that will keep it in balance. If you are having a difficult time with your food choices, portions, and so on, maybe put some thought into the idea that your body craves whichever state of balance it is currently in. If it's not in the right state, slowly introduce foods to move it to a better state. Once there, it will continue to *want* to stay in it.

If you are not in need of actual therapy or counseling for food behaviors, the goal is different. Instead, you will want to create behavior patterns that lead to a more consistent way of handling the relationship to food. Building a consistent practice in your life with the approach to every level of your healing is always the goal. If you feel led to try certain diets, be sure that you are doing so mindfully. Get your blood tested before and after trying to find a way to eat that works best for you. Try not to get pulled in with fad diets. Instead try to find a practice with food that can be lifelong and well maintained. Jumping from diet to diet can wreak havoc on your body. Balance is the goal with all of this. Be careful and be mindful.

⌘ Practice: Food Awareness

Take out a journal and document how often you eat and what you eat. With each offering of food and time of day, also make a note of how you are feeling or if anything has you emotionally charged up when choosing particular foods. For the best results, track a minimum of three days. Notice your habits and sit with them to determine your eating style and if you are happy with what you see. Food changes begin with becoming aware of our patterns, so seeing them in black and white can be pretty eye-opening. Remember not to judge *what* you eat; you are just documenting your choices and habits so you can make decisions that will help you create a healthy approach to what you eat and why.

2. Sleep

The second pillar for optimum wellness is in getting adequate sleep. So few of us seem to get enough rest, despite the abundance of information out there about it. Sleep affects not only our physical bodies but our emotional regulators as well. Our body clock, also known as our circadian rhythm, regulates our bodily functions. Interestingly enough, there is a main body clock located in the hypothalamus of the brain, as well as other minor body clocks located in the tissues of the body peripherally. These little clocks rearrange themselves as needed according to natural light.[3]

3. Frank Scheer, "Circadian Rhythms: How Irregular Sleep Patterns Impact Your Health." Brigham Health Hub https://brighamhealthhub.org/healthy-living/circadian-rhythms-how-irregular-sleep-patterns-impact-your-health.

When a person gets adequate rest for a specified length of time on a regular basis, the body works to repair itself of many physical ailments. Adequate rest also has a huge impact on a person's emotional stability. How short-tempered do we tend to be when we have not been resting well? Being sleep deprived can make people more emotionally reactive or even cause negative thoughts and behaviors. It can lead to anxiety and a disconnect between the self and loved ones.

Sleep affects every part of life and is super important. But doesn't it seem that how much sleep we are able to get changes during different times in our lives? If you are currently in a place (say, with young children or acting as a caregiver) where sleep isn't so easy to get, be gentle with yourself and understand that sleep patterns do change as the parameters of your life changes. For this section, my offering is this:

1. Sleep is at the top of the list of importance for health and repair of the physical and emotional bodies.

2. Take a rest anytime you get the opportunity.

3. Be mindful of your moods, behaviors, and temper if sleep hasn't been your friend.

4. See a doctor if your sleep patterns are really wonky (or if you might need adjustments such as a CPAP machine due to sleep apnea).

5. Work within your allotted sleep patterns. Because I sleep in waves, I acknowledge that the first part of the night is where I get my deepest and best sleep. I take advantage of it. I give thanks for it and ask politely for Spirit to please give me some more of where that came from.

6. When I can't sleep, I pray. I spend a lot of time in the night in prayer, contemplation, and meditation. I get my best conversations in with Spirit in the wee hours of the night. I try not to waste the time where I'm finding myself in between the sleep and waking states. This is also the time where I get up and write when I've been woken by Spirit for creative purposes, which happens to me a great deal. Spirit wakes me to get up, listen, and write their wisdom. When Spirit comes knocking, I follow the flow, no matter what time it is.

7. You might have waking sleep patterns because Spirit is lively in the dark hours of the night. Pay attention to when and why you might not be sleeping all the way

through or waking up still exhausted. Sometimes even when you've been sleeping you wake exhausted, one possible reason is that you've been astral traveling outside of your body all night long. If you are not sleeping restoratively, check on yourself and figure out where to go. Ask yourself the right questions and answer honestly for best results.

⌘ Practice: Getting to Sleep

Before you lie down for the night, be sure that you have completed any tasks that might keep you up thinking about them. Every person has a different nighttime ritual, and some work better than others. Try not to drink liquids too close to bed time as well. Ideally, you are able to sleep uninterrupted throughout the night. Being mindful about your sleep practice is only going to help you. Clear your mind, clear your space, and prepare yourself to enter a deep sleep. Either listen to a guided meditation to help you sleep. (In our home, we listen to my own guided sleep meditation created with a hypnotherapist to help put us into REM sleep. See the additional recommended resources for a link to this meditation.)

Clear the mind by gently focusing on your breath. Take a nice, easy breath in through your nose and a long exhale through the mouth. Repeat this pattern until your body begins to follow naturally. Go through your body and notice whether you are holding any tension. Feel your feet and let them fall apart. Notice your hands—are they open and relaxed or are you holding in a clenched fist? Pay attention to your mouth and face muscles. Let your jaw relax, and don't let the top and bottom teeth touch. Rather, allow them to be slightly separated and relaxed. The tongue can rest gently against the roof or the bottom of the mouth, never pushing against the teeth. As you relax each part of your body, ask it to let go. Doing so will save you some time in falling into a deeper sleep. People sometimes shake and jolt as they enter dreamtime, which I believe is due to the incredible amounts of tension the body has to wade through in order to let go enough to sleep. Set your intention to sleep deeply and peacefully and wake rested and energized.

3. Stress Control

The third pillar for optimum wellness is how we choose to handle stressors in our lives. While we can't really control the things around us unless we are removed from everything entirely, it is possible to control the way in which we choose to react. I took a friend to my naturopath for NAET treatment (Nambrudipad's Allergy Elimination Technique), which is used for a number of things, but to be brief, is like a reboot for the body's various systems to be less sensitive to various elements. My naturopath first did a muscle test and then went deeper into whether the issue is physical, emotional, environmental, or something else. This friend had some trauma to the brain left over from a collision several years back that left him with an epilepsy diagnosis that included extremely difficult seizures.[4] After the tests, the naturopath showed my friend how totally different his strength was when his brain was tested versus when his stressed brain was tested. This is one of those times where I wish I could post a video to show the night and day difference in his brain strength when stress entered the picture. On their own, my friend's test results were strong. The damage (for him and many of us) came from the stress patterns he had been working under. Stress is no joke, and we don't do a great job truly articulating just how powerful of a force it is.

As a culture, we are aware that stress is rampant but also have collectively learned how to desensitize ourselves to it and work around it instead. We ignore the stress patterns we've put in place for ourselves that stem from years of denial and lack of awareness. It is dangerous to our well-being in every way. Learning to work with your body/mind to calm yourself when faced with an overwhelming stimulus is truly one of the greatest coping skills you can possibly arm yourself with. Taking little breaks out from whatever is happening is a big ticket to healing that I'm handing you right now.

Many times, the things that stress us aren't really even about us at all. First, size up any given situation and ask, "Is this even my stuff? What happens if I make no choice? Am I going out of my way to insert myself into something that isn't necessary? Am I overreacting? Am I being overly sensitive?" If there is tension between you and someone else, it can be easier to nip when you approach with honesty of how something made you feel. Being

---

4. Jeffrey Englander, David X. Cifu, Ramon Diaz-Arrastia, "Seizures after Traumatic Brain Injury" *Archives of Physical Medicine and Rehabilitation* June 2014 95(6): 1223–1224. https://www.ncbi.nlm.nih.gov/pmc/articles/PMC4516165/.

vulnerable and honest about something that caused you emotional distress usually shuts the other person down when approached with sincerity. People aren't used to others being so open and honest, so it quickly diffuses the situation. Things like "It hurt my feelings and embarrassed me when you said this to me in front of other people," or "I'm sorry I lashed out at you. I felt angry when you said this to me and instead of saying it hurt me, I behaved in a way that sounded angry when really I was hurt." The words *I'm sorry* are powerful and can end things quickly. Learning to become more honest in the moment with your feelings is a huge stress reducer. You won't have to go home and stew over things for days while raising those stress levels up higher. Reevaluating any given situation that brings about stress can offer real strength in your emotional game. Do whatever you can to keep things as stress free and light hearted as possible without taking it on the chin. When you are caught in a situation that needs your attention, you have a choice to make about how you will carry on. You can face it head on one last time, or you can simply walk away.

"You always have a choice" used to bother me as a statement because there were some situations where it seemed like that wasn't true. Some people come with the package even if you didn't choose for them to be part of your web of life. However, the truth is (and it can be hard to hear) that you do always have a choice whether to remove yourself from certain people or situations, but it will likely come with a price. If something doesn't feed your soul, why are you sitting at that table? Get up and go sit somewhere else. You can remove yourself whenever you choose. The kicker is that until it's done without attachment to the outcome, it will not be a permanent removal.

I remember a friend's boyfriend made a comment many years ago that applies to this idea. He said that if she loved him, this was a good thing. If she hated him, this too could still be a good thing because then he still had a chance to win her back. Love and hate share a very fine line, as they are both places of passion that are filled with attachments. It wasn't dislike but indifference that would really let him know for sure that she would be out of his life forever. When you don't have any attachment to the person or the outcome, then you will find freedom. If you can remove yourself from any stressful component, situation or person, do your best to do so without an attachment to how they feel, how they react, what they say, and so on. They can talk smack about you to everyone that will listen, but it won't mean anything to you anymore. Your liberation is born in the place where your decision no longer meets with the "requirement" that you need approval to leave. It can rearrange everything in your world when you remove yourself from the expectations of the outcomes.

⌘ Practice: Lessen Stress

When things become overwhelming or you find that you are not able to let go of your thoughts, take a step back and sit out for a moment. Close your eyes and exhale fully before taking a slow, deep inhale in through your nose and exhale out through the mouth. For the next ten breaths inhale one single word that you want to bring into your body. For the next ten exhales release one single word or thought that you want out of your space. Here are some examples:

- Inhale love, exhale fear.
- Inhale calm, exhale frustration.
- Inhale tranquility, exhale rage.
- Inhale vacation, exhale (name of someone driving you nuts!)

Make the practice personal to you; it's not a bad thing to let go of someone who treats you poorly or makes you crazy. Notice how much better it feels without that person or thought and hang on to it! Then start to notice the softer and more positive words you came up with. This exercise can be a big indicator of the things you most love and want and the things you most want to get away from.

4. Attitude/Mindset

The fourth pillar for optimum wellness is keeping a proper mindset. For best emotional health, we must address our mental attitude toward ourselves and others. It's simple but it's true. Taking an attitude of gratitude will free you. If you can learn to notice the little things and appreciate them more, you'll make room to continue to appreciate the bigger things. Before you know it, so much new room opens up in your mind. When I was in the throes of anxiety and panic, it was extremely difficult to give thanks for anything at all—I didn't notice a single thing outside of myself and my strange symptoms. Somewhere in it, I began to listen to all those people talk about being grateful for the simple little things. I began to expand my own vision and awareness. I began to give thanks every night for the day and every morning for the night. I began to give thanks for the food, the company, and the roof over my head. Even when that meant me crashing on a friend's pullout couch, it didn't matter. Once you begin to be thankful it multiplies and becomes something entirely new.

I try to live my life in constant gratitude. Though some people find it annoying, others are curious about it and want to learn themselves. Many friends have asked me how in the world I got so happy. What was my secret? Is it even real? I tell them that it *is* real—I am truly very happy and do my best to live from a state of constant gratitude. I notice things that I used to take for granted. I love being alive and I love life! I love just being able to close my eyes and listen to my own breathing and be grateful for them. It isn't fake. I am truly so blessed. When I get off track and take for granted the incredible miracles and gifts I've received in this life, I back up and reevaluate until I see more of it. I step into my grateful space. Nothing is perfect and nothing was ever meant to be. I am keenly aware of just how wonderful life has become and do not belittle the amount of work I've put into myself and my life to make this happen. It takes work daily to continue and keep showing up for yourself. It takes courage to allow yourself to be happy. I know that sounds silly, but it's true. It's easier to slump down and assume the worst. It's harder and requires more tenacity to be open for the very best to see what the Universe is willing to offer each day. Looking at things—negatively or positively—is a habit. Some of us learned it from our parents and some from our peers. At this point, however, it does not matter where it was learned; it only matters that you change it now.

Here is what I know to be true: the Universe will match your perception of reality. You can have the very best life right now if you will allow yourself to do so. You must show up and be open to receive and know you are worth all the sunshiny sparkles the world has to offer. *You are worth every penny in the Universe, my friend. And so am I.*

⌘ Practice: Affirmations

Following are seven affirmations, one for each day of the week. Once you do all seven, you can repeat or write your own. After you get started, you will want to keep up the practice. Look at yourself in the mirror when you say these affirmations and repeat them as often as you are able throughout the day.

1. I am free to be happy and choose how I'm going to feel today.
2. I am strong, capable, and smart.

3. I know what I know, and I know it confidently.

4. Today, I choose kindness to myself and everyone around me.

5. I AM a badass.

6. The light inside me is free to shine and sparkle.

7. Today I choose to be comfortable in my skin. I love myself. I am LOVE.

5. Movement

The fifth pillar for wellness is movement; I can't ignore the physical bodily movement component, whether it's dance, kickboxing, martial arts, yoga, walking, running, water aerobics, Sufi dancing, or bowling. I don't have any judgments about how you choose to move your body and increase your health—just do it! It's important that what you choose to do is something that you actually *enjoy* instead of something you make yourself do. Remember to have a "want to do" approach, not a "have to do" one. An exercise practice is paramount for moving energy and releasing whatever is not serving your best self. When we have too much energy and it has no place to go, it becomes overwhelming. We need to release it through writing, drawing, expressing, and moving. Our bodies must have a part in the rearranging of energy within ourselves. It's so much easier to get moving when you've already been moving. To paraphrase Newton's first law of motion, a body that is already moving with exercise will stay moving with exercise. The body that decided to stop all movement and sit will have a hard time getting back into motion. I've been both in my life: super-high, nonstop motion and total dead weight. Becoming active again is one of the hardest things we can do but also one of the most rewarding. We all deserve to live happy, healthy, well-balanced lives, so we have to be willing to do the work required to create and maintain them. These are not situations that happen *to* us, they happen *with* us. Up or down, active or still, we made a decision. Because we have the power, we can unmake it and re-decide in any given moment.

✤ PRACTICE: BEGIN MOVING

Start small—do something that makes you giggle. The internet is full of videos of dance moves and songs you can follow. Even if you are with your kids, you can visit gonoodle.com and find a funny song to dance to (with instructions). Do one song every day for ten days (it does not have to be the same song or dance) to see if it helps you get motivated to do more. If this offering doesn't work for you, go outside and take a walk. And while you're walking, ask yourself what you've got against dancing!

The Rest of What's to Come

Now that we've looked at the body as an integrated whole and the ways in which we can set ourselves up for healing, let's take a deeper look at the various body layers individually. When it comes to being healthy or becoming a healthier version of yourself, hopefully here you will find the tools necessary to understand everything involved. As mentioned in the introduction, I wrote this book in the hopes that when something feels off, you will have enough information to pause to pinpoint which aspect of the body needs focus and possibly who to go to for help. For example, maybe you call your naturopath or homeopath and undergo a test for heavy metals. You may end up working with a dietician, nutritionist, or holistic practitioner to create a specific diet. It might be that your energy is off, so visiting an acupuncturist or seeing an Ayurvedic practitioner is the key. Maybe you have physical pain and need to see a chiropractor for an adjustment. Perhaps you notice that you feel depressed or anxious and know it's time to find a therapist.

The best thing you can do is become so in tune with your body that you can hear its call whenever it becomes out of balance. It's crucial to be able to interpret that out-of-balance feeling as soon as it occurs so that you can tune in and find out what may be off, as is having faith that there is always an answer and there is always another way. Work with your body systems and the right team to find your path through it all—it is your greatest treasure. I hope you always listen to your own instincts. If it feels right in your gut, go for it. If you feel a sense of trepidation, trust that too. Question why you might be holding back, and trust your answers. Become your best advocate for whole body health and wellness. This is your life, so it's up to you to make it what you want it to be. Take charge of the world around you and the part you are playing in it.

Trust that when you tap into yourself and your connection to the Universe, the next best step will be provided. You don't have to have the whole plan; you just have to keep doing the single steps. Keep checking your gut and dialoguing with your spirit team. Keep them close and never forget to give thanks and acknowledgment. Together you will navigate your way into wholeness.

Part II
The Physical Body

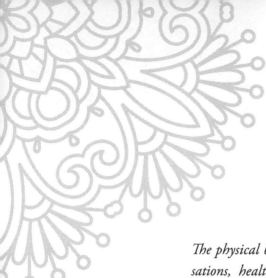

The physical body is where you experience all of the earthly sensations, healthy and painful. With the right mindset, proper research, and the willingness to think both inside and outside the box, you can become a healthier and greatly enhanced version of yourself. I have supreme faith in your ability to shift and heal. Your best life is waiting for you to claim it and step fully into it. Don't be afraid to get messy.

Chapter 3
Getting Started

Learning to differentiate which aspect of the body we need to gather information on is the first step to identifying the issue and creating a plan of action. When it comes to the physical body, this pertains to every part of our physical beings. In this chapter we will begin navigating our way through our physical bodies. We will also learn how to gather proper data and/or a diagnosis to help establish a game plan for this area.

The first item of business when approaching any shift in healing is to collect our data. If something is affecting the physical body, you must first define the situation and get concrete facts to back it up. If it is a disease, illness, sickness, or issue (from most intense to least), first find out for certain exactly what it is you are dealing with. A proper defining or diagnosis of the issue is paramount to making the correct first steps in the right direction, even though the task can be daunting. If you need to obtain a diagnosis, the process will likely and hopefully include tests, X-rays, scans, fluid samples, and so on. So many people fit into the camp of not really knowing for sure what the diagnosis even is. Because there are so many false positive and false negative results out there, always seek a second opinion (or more if you need to). If you have an issue and not an illness (e.g., an emotional situation that has gotten to be too difficult to manage alone), it might not require a specific diagnosis through physical testing but may still require a specific definition or diagnosis laid out by a different professional. It may be a cognitive therapist, a spiritual counselor, or any range of practitioners from the alternative, regenerative, functional, or integrative medical side. This is the time to seek someone who is wise and practiced, not friends or coaches. Diagnostics come in many forms. Be open to all through the specific intended avenues necessary to obtain your correct starting point.

Next, we need to center, get on the same team within ourselves, and clearly define our intentions. And to define our intentions, we must go back to answering the big three questions in the previous chapter. Only after this can we collect and assemble our outside team: a medical team, alternative healing team, spirit team, and any cheerleaders (the people you surround yourself with who are helpful in your healing).

Before we begin, please know that magic and miracles can happen at any time along this path. It is most important to be open to this concept. Look wide, search far, and trust your inner guidance. Your soul always knows the way.

The physical body is where we feel the experiences of our bodies being healthy or not. It is also the place from where we need to collect the most data to make decisions. This is the layer of ourselves that likely requires medical teams—our primary care doctor and any specialists if needed. We need doctors who have their finger on the pulse of the latest research according to their field and who are willing to listen to and work with us.

The next step after finding out your true starting point is the other big-ticket item: research. When engaging in research, you must be willing to look at both sides of the aisle. Research should be all-encompassing—*much* more than just looking on the internet! As well, it's more than just meeting with doctors, sharing with friends, and asking for advice or stories others have heard. All of these things are part of research, but there's much more. Research could also be opening yourself up in a way you have never done before in order to find as much information as possible. Search for it and find it from any place it comes.

Not every answer will be at your current medical provider's office, though it's equally as true that you'll receive important information there, so stay open to all information that comes your way.

There Is Always Another Way

The three most researched and practiced medical systems used throughout the world are Western medicine, Chinese Medicine, and Ayurevedic medicine. Each of these approaches to health care is vastly different from the others and therefore offer totally unique approaches to prevention, recovery, and health. Just because you might only be familiar with one approach does not negate the validity of the others. People jump on a plane and fly across the world to save their lives when they may have exhausted all efforts of the health care local to their area. So when I discuss research, I'm asking that you look beyond the one scope you've been told to look at for healing. Each of the different ways of approaching the body carry with it hundreds to thousands of years of research and discovery.

Here is what I know to be true: *there is always another way.* There is always an alternative approach to healing that can put you in the same end game as another approach. One is not uniformly better; one works better for you personally. The task is to find that route if the first one isn't working. Does this mean that a holistic approach or the Western medical approach are the only way, and you should disregard anything else? Definitely not. With the right diagnosis and correct information, you can go down *both* paths simultaneously—the "straight" one that is prescribed and customarily offered and the alternate route that might be a bit more esoteric and unusual. One does not take away from the other. More times than not, you need both in order to get long-lasting, life-changing results. I believe incorporating healing opportunities beyond the standard protocol of anything is where recovery lives, more so than simply getting to the place where things are simply manageable.

There is always some sort of help, answer, treatment, or opportunity that may be what saves you or a loved one's life. An alternative route exists somewhere. It is up to you to find the best avenues for your healing, wherever that may take you. People who live in other countries pack up their stuff and come to this country for treatments that are not offered in their countries just as people in our country pack up and head out to places to do the same. Why? Because there is always another avenue for healing. Understand that there is no implication that the answers to your healing live across the world. A certain treatment that you find that is from another part of the world might have practitioners right down the road from you once you start searching for them. Willingness and curiosity separate the survivors from the thrivers, and my vote is always for all of us to thrive.

The Matchmaker

I pride myself on being a really great matchmaker for two things:

1. Animals: I can put a dog or cat with the right people or family. It's an instinct, and I do it well.

2. Healing: I can put people on a healing path with fantastic options of who to see for their healing. People tell me what's going on, and I sit with it for a bit and then feel in my gut where they need to go to help them along their path. I am not a medical intuitive, but I am intuitive when it comes to health and healing options that I believe could be beneficial.

A friend I met in yoga class told me that she suffers greatly from a spinal condition called ankylosing spondylitis for which she's been on medication for more than a decade. I suggested she see a craniosacral therapist as well as a local acupuncturist who is a retired neurologist from Beijing. It turned out that the acupuncturist did not think the condition was the correct diagnosis and instead believed it to be neurological. He then sent her to a neurological specialist who diagnosed her with migraines—she didn't have the spinal issue at all! With this correct diagnosis, they were able to treat her easily and with much milder treatments. She told me at class that thanks to my suggestion, she found the correct issue and treatment and now is off the meds for the spondylitis. She is now on a medication for the migraines that works fast and stops the three-day flare-ups she had always believed to be spondylitis flares. Now she can move and practice yoga without the constant pain. This is a simple example of how getting the proper diagnosis and treatment is the most important step in any healing process. Everyone makes their decisions on health and healing based on their own experiences and belief systems, and doctors are no different. Be mindful of who you are seeing for your issues and know that you might need to visit more than one specialist to confirm a diagnosis.

If you are faced with needing to heal something big, be willing to move outside of the belief systems you or those around you have set for you and be willing to look through a much wider lens into what is possible. Put it in steps as you determine your best plan for health and healing. Remember that the process goes both ways: when it comes to anyone else's healing choices, it is not your right to judge another's approach to their health and healing either.

When a very close family member was diagnosed with breast cancer, I was speaking with a respected elder and confided in him what was going on. I said that given the triple negative markers (meaning the cancer was multiplying at a fast-acting pace), my family member had decided to forgo the lumpectomy and go for a radical double mastectomy. His response to me was, "You are not going to let them cut into her, are you? Those surgeons are butchers!" While I appreciated his two cents, I also had great respect for my family member for being so brave and doing what it took to save her life. Had I turned on her and decided the elder was right and surgeons are nothing but butchers, I could not have been the support person she needed me to be. Imagine if I had acted in a behavior consistent with the opinions of someone else and taken them on as my own. Instead, I was in that chemo suite for every appointment, and I emptied her drains after surgery three times a day. I was the one she leaned on and needed as her support person. I was blown away by her strength and conviction. She saved her own life by making that decision, and she was quick about it too. She didn't hesitate. She told the surgeon what they were going to do, and she wanted to do it the following week.

If whoever you saw today doesn't have the answers you need, do not stop there. Go find someone else, another practitioner from another narrative of diagnostics. Search out further and wider and find someone who specializes in the part of your body you need information about. Your body is your temple, so you must take charge of whatever might be happening within it. Essential to this process is knowing where you are starting from, which is where Western allopathic methods belong, whether in the form of a proper diagnosis that can only be known through the avenues of proper testing, scans, blood or lab work, or something clinical. Never take anyone's word for what you might be experiencing without anything to back it up. We have to be a part of this process. If you get a diagnosis (or worse, a guess) that doesn't feel right, do not stop. Go seek another opinion. If my doctors or specialists can't find an answer, I keep knocking on the healing doors until I find the answers that resonate with me. To put it another way, you could go to five doctors who specialize in the same field and get five different answers for your health. Tests are definitive, but the treatments and other options are the result of each individual's knowledge and instincts. It is therefore crucial to line up with those that best fit your needs. If the first approach doesn't resonate, keep looking. Even the medical field is full of contradictions. We are all human doing the best we can with what we've got.

Research

The research part of any healing journey is as important as finding the right diagnosis. Facts are necessary for giving us the starting point that we need in order to create our best route to healing. However, are facts really our friends? In this day and age, we must understand a few things. First, even in scientific research, whoever is doing the research can skew the science and testing to support their initial hypothesis. Research can be very biased. We need to understand that there are different types of research that mean different things, and so what we look for when reading it will be different too. The other part of any research you need to ask and find out is, who funded this particular research? It is a proven fact that many of the research links and arguments for certain illnesses were funded by the companies who created the medicine for it, a practice that is so common (and dangerous) in our world because these companies bank on the fact that you don't know any better and take all the research and findings at face value. It's often that we don't find out until it's much too late that the research was funded through those pharmaceutical companies with potentially skewed results. Not enough people know to follow up with a scrutiny that is worthy of such research offerings. Questions to consider when looking at any research:

1. Who did the funding?
2. Who did the research?
3. Does any research exist with double-blind or peer-reviewed studies? (and what do those things even mean?)

At this stage (on the physical layer), it is important to do some fact-checking about an illness, its diagnosis, and any possible treatments, so be sure you come into any research knowing what to really look for in your findings. Until someone pointed these things out to me and I studied them in my graduate program at my university, I had no idea how wide and varied research really is. It wasn't until I went back to school that I learned to ask question such as, "Is it peer reviewed?" and "Can it be proven?" And it was through the autism community that I learned to question who was behind research in the first place. How was it funded? Which doctors were chosen for the studies, and who do those doctors work for? Those questions are very important to answer before you make a decision about early treatment.

Let's define these research elements so you know better what to search for. I'm going to simplify each one of the terms affiliated with studies. Why is this important to know? Because if you do have any particular illness and you are doing your research and you come across a shot or pill that looks like it's going to work for you, you must know where those studies have come from and who funded them. Too many times studies are bought and paid for by the medical companies or their doctors, or the research was not conducted objectively with double-blind controls or placebos.

Blind study: One party in the research is in the know of the testing procedures and the person being tested is not. These can be very misleading and biased. Be careful with blind studies.

Double-blind study: Both the tester and the subject are blinded to the testing process. This is the best environment for fairness in research.

Peer-reviewed study: After reviewing the initial findings or studies conducted, other doctors, researchers, or people in the same field approve the quality or competence of the initial findings. You can find examples in scholarly research sites such as googlescholar .com, pubmed.com, and scholarly journals. These are more trustworthy sources.

Meta-analysis: Research from several different studies and resources is pulled and collected in a single report. Some people love meta-analysis because of the wide range of research in one place, while others prefer a more concrete single study.

Placebo studies: When a study group takes whatever product or ingredient is being tested and another group thinks they are taking the same product but in actuality are taking something like a sugar pill or another option that is fake. The groups don't know which product they actually received, and therefore the results are unbiased.

The most honest and fair research is published in scholarly journals in the same field. However, this does *not* mean that the research was not funded by companies with a serious interest in the results of said studies. Again, you need to keep looking into the research to figure out what is being presented and how it got there.

Research and Funding

This is the tricky grey area for research, and it can bite you if you let it. If the research is government-funded, then by law any literature must list who provided the funding for the studies. However, if the research is privately funded (as is the case with so many pharmaceutical research studies), they are not required by law to disclose who was funding the research. Companies who have a vested interest in the results generally hire their own team of experts to lead the studies and do not disclose that they are behind it. Once published, they are quick to put it out everywhere and call it fact. When you are doing your own research to find medical answers for yourself or a loved one, you must be extremely skeptical when reading research.

Research the pros, research the cons. Research the allopathic Western medical side, research the traditional Eastern medical side, and try your best to research beyond both. Find stories of people who have done amazing things in the realm of what you yourself need in order to restore balance to your system. Find out how they did it. You cannot afford to be narrow-minded in your search or stop after the first result.

Alternative Research

This is the part about research where I take you away from the funding, testing, and scholarly articles. Now we shift your attention and focus to reviews from actual people who have received treatments. Peer-reviewed research is valuable, but the main purpose of it is usually publication. Reviews from real people who have used the products or received the treatments hold considerable weight when you are searching for your next steps on your journey

However, the phrase "alternative research" does not allude to alternative truths. Instead, it leans to a negative bias toward certain treatments either because not enough laboratory testing has been able to prove the efficacy or because a lot of holistic or herbal treatments are not recognized by the regulatory agencies and therefore are assumed to be bunk. Many times, science is late on the findings. Keep an open mind to hearing personal experiences, as they might serve you well.

Just because a product or treatment has not been academically or formally vetted does not mean it is not highly effective or healthy. I'm going to contradict what I said earlier on research and say that it's my personal perception that not everything on the Quackwatch website deserves to be there. For example, NAET (Nambudripad's Allergy Elimination Technique, which is covered later on) appears as a Quackwatch result.[5] However, I have recently found research-based articles published in medical and scholarly journals stating NAET's effectiveness.[6] For myself as well as my family, it has been one of the strongest

---

5. Stephen Barrett, "Applied Kinesiology: Phony Muscle-Testing for 'Allergies' and 'Nutrient Deficiencies.'" https://www.quackwatch.org/01QuackeryRelatedTopics/Tests/ak.html.

6. Caroline B. Terwee, "Successful treatment of food allergy with Nambudripad's Allergy Elimination Techniques (NAET) in a 3-year-old: A Case Report," September 19, 2008. Doi: 10.1186/1757-1626-1-166.

and most beneficial treatments in our arsenal for healing every person in my family for various issues.

Research, Review, and Trust

Here is where we add the third component to the first two (gather your facts and information, and research every angle in which to find the avenues that will offer healing, respectively): tap into your Divine inner wisdom to figure out which move to make. Gather, look, listen, and move. Going with your gut is the movement part of the equation. Figuring out which way to move is through the inner wisdom responses. You cannot do this alone—no one can. From here, your action will be about tapping into the higher source to guide you to each next best step in your healing journey.

⌘ Practice: The Body Scan

Every morning we need to start our day with a quick check-in with our body to determine how we are feeling and where we are at. Feel your body with your mind, starting from your feet and working all the way through the stations: ankles, knees, hips, stomach/gut, chest, low back, spine, whole back, shoulders, arms, elbows, wrists, hands, neck, ears, mouth, nose, chin, cheeks, forehead, eyes, scalp of the head. Is anything feeling off? Does any place hurt? Does it feel tight or sore anywhere? When you go to the bathroom, are all systems go? While small, these are basic things that need attention. Remember that little things that go ignored can easily become the bigger things, so pay attention to every part of your body. If you answered yes to "Does anything hurt," look more deeply into that answer. Where does it hurt? Why does it hurt? Is it surface level or might it be deeper, like in an organ? Is it a bruise or is something happening? Can you pinpoint the exact location or is it an area? Should you call your doctor and have it looked at? These are extremely important things to ask yourself. If your answer is "I probably should call my doctor but can't afford it/don't want to deal with it/don't have time for it/don't really care," these are also important things to note! Next we go into a different set of questions: "Is this something with my mood, emotions, or mind?" "Am I feeling disconnected from myself and my body? Am I possibly feeling depressed or anxious?" Look into these answers as well and see if you have the same four responses as above. And after you've had your wake-up time maybe within an hour of waking, ask the really important question that might take care of all the rest: Are you hungry? Have you eaten? When was the last time you ate? So many times, we are moody, cranky, disconnected, or agitated ("hangry," as they call it) if our blood sugar is not balanced. Simplistic as they might sound, the body scan and check-in are important tools in your arsenal that need to be used every single day. Our bodies are master communicators, so it's high time we start learning how to listen! Make notes to yourself if something comes up so that you don't shrug it off as something insignificant. You can't track information if it's not ever catalogued. Maybe do a hand-written journal or a spreadsheet on your computer—just something on the side to note symptoms and situations that arise during your scans.

I hope this chapter expanded your horizons on research—what it can be and what it might not be. I hope that it got you practicing your body scan daily and really beginning to tune in on a deeper level within your physical body. Ignoring little symptoms here and there can lead to big issues with time. It's up to each of us to be on top of our own game. That starts here.

Chapter 4
The Physical Body Defined

In this chapter we will concentrate on the physical self and how it functions in relation to the whole. The matters related to this topic range from very basic to more detailed information we just barely understand. Outlined and detailed in this chapter are the physical body, skin, bone, tissue, blood/plasma, muscles, fascia, nerves, and organs. Everyone should have a basic foundation of knowledge regarding their bodies and what's in them.

The physical body is only one layer of our bodies, though it is the densest and most primary layer, consisting of everything from our skin inward. If something is off within our bodies, it is most appropriate to see the doctor and undergo standard medical practices for an accurate diagnosis. It is in this space that we need to gather solid information based entirely on facts, tests, scans, blood work, and so on. If you need specific and definitive answers, accept nothing less than a specialist. Now is not the time to go to the general doctor and accept guesses for your answers. Note as well that doctors of specialties only work within one of the eleven body systems. Keeping this in mind will help you define who to see for what reason, should you need them. The following is a list of a physiological system, a brief description of what it entails, as well as the doctors and alternative approaches within the same scope.

Specialists According to Body Systems

There are eleven body systems categorized by specialties in medical practice. They are as follows:

1. Respiratory system: This covers the trachea and lungs. The specialist who falls under this category is a pulmonologist. A pulmonologist works with the lungs and pulmonary disorders such as COPD and pneumonia.

2. Nervous system: This system is composed of the brain and spinal cord. A neurologist is considered the specialist for brain and nerve issues. Other practitioners who work with this element include a chiropractor, who helps with spine and nerve issues including many other ailments. A craniosacral therapist also works with this system and is who I credit for my child's recovery through her autism diagnosis. An acupuncturist can also treat many disorders that involve the nervous system.

3. Endocrine system: This is the group of glands that regulate our body processes such as reproduction, growing, and how our body absorbs and uses nutrients from food. The glands of the endocrine system are the pituitary gland, the pineal gland, the thyroid, thymus, adrenal glands, and pancreas. Endocrinologists work with hormone balancing, diabetes, thyroid disorders, and with any other glandular or hormonal imbalances.

4. Circulatory system: This system is what circulates the blood throughout the body. The heart, veins, and arteries make up this body system. A cardiologist (heart and vascular disorders), vascular surgeons (training in blood vessels and surgery) are the related specialists.

5. Skeletal system: This is the bones, ligaments, tendons, muscles, and nerves. An orthopedic doctor/surgeon will diagnose and likely perform surgery within this body system. Osteopath physicians work with joints, muscles, and the spine. They treat through their own hands a patient's bones and body alignment. For bone disorders like osteoporosis, several can treat and diagnose including internists (doctors of internal medicine), gynecologists, rheumatologists, endocrinologists, and geriatric doctors. On the recovery side of surgery, broken bones see a physical therapist (PT).

6. Lymphatic system: This is your body's plumbing system that is in charge of waste removal. The system is a network of vessels that drain from the tissues into the blood. Lymphatic and immune disease doctors include the lymphologist, hematologist, and oncologist (who works using radiology to get diagnostics on the lymphatic system). A lymphocintegram can be ordered through any of these

specialists to determine where in the lymph vessels an obstruction may exist. For treatment of the body with swelling issues, or a chronic condition called lymphedema, a manual lymphatic drainage therapist with combined decongestive therapy training is key.

7. Reproductive system: The reproductive system covers the sex organs. For men, the doctor to help with issues in this area is a urologist, who can help identify and treat cancers that occur in the urinary tract, prostate, issues within the penis, vasectomies or reversals, as well as kidney stones. For women, the doctor is an OB-GYN, or obstetrics-gynecologist, who provides the testing and treatments for the female reproductive system. If you are of the age where you are considering bearing children or have already had children, the preferred doctor would be an obstetrician, a gynecologist who specializes in care for women before, during, and after childbirth.

8. Renal system: This system includes urinary, excretory, and bladder/kidney function. A urologist works with urine, bladder, and kidney issues as well as vasectomy surgery (see above). A nephrologist specializes in kidney and renal care.

9. Integumentary system: In this system are the hair, nails, skin, and sweat. Dermatologists treat all things skin-related, as well as hair, nails, and skin cancers. If the issue is skin-related but not in need of a doctor, see an esthetician. They are skin-care specialists who work with the face, neck, head, arms, and shoulders. For sweat issues (the term is *hyperhidrosis* for excessive sweating), doctors who can treat this condition include: family medicine, primary care, internists, and neurologists.

10. Digestive system: This system covers the full digestive and gastrointestinal tract that includes the teeth, tongue, esophagus, stomach, small and large intestines, salivary glands, liver, gallbladder, and pancreas. A gastroenterologist can treat and work with issues such as: Crohn's disease, irritable bowel syndrome (IBS), heartburn, acid reflux, digestive issues, and GERD (gastroesophageal reflux disease).

11. Muscular system: For muscular issues, the specialists to see are orthopedic doctors of sports-medicine practices, either orthopedic surgeon or primary care physicians who works with athletes. Rheumatologists treat muscles, tendons, joints, bones, osteoarthritis, and rheumatoid arthritis. Physical therapists work with the whole body in recovering and restoring strength and balance. Massage therapists work with the muscles as well. Massage practices vary far and wide; clinical, neuromuscular, deep tissue, myofascial release, myoskeletal release, in

addition to many others offer help with muscle issues. For practicioners who work with the fascia, a basic list includes craniosacral therapists, myoskeletal therapists, orthopedic massage practitioners, myofascial therapists, acupuncturists, cryotherapists, or specialists who teach stretching, tai chi, qi gong, and yoga.

Seeking Out a Professional Touch

The following specialists work with various parts of the body, but their practice often includes overlaps of two or more of the body's eleven systems and are therefore in their own category here.

Massage Therapy: While not everyone enjoys bodywork, it is important to know what is out there if you are not familiar. There is a chart on massage therapy in the appendix for bodywork specialties for soft tissue. Massage therapy and bodywork can help you with a host of issues beyond needing to relax. If you haven't ever received a treatment and think it's only for the wealthy, there are plenty of ways to get the work you need. Call the local massage school and schedule appointments with their clinic for services—the price is always discounted, and the teachers and students pay special care in your treatment. If there are parts of the body nothing else has helped with, please look over the chart and see if there is a service offered that you hadn't thought of before. From there, follow the road map about doing your research. Go with your gut on who to see for what treatment you are seeking.

Ears/Otolaryngology: Ear, nose, and throat doctors (formally known as otolaryngologists) work with disorders of the ears, nose, throat, head, and neck. Other alternative practice for the ears would be auricular therapy or ear acupuncture a trained acupuncturist can perform for assessment and treatment of overall body health through the specific points on the ears.

Eyes/Vision: For eye-related issues, an optometrist or an ophthalmologist would be the specialists to visit. An optometrist can check the vision and can prescribe corrective lenses, while ophthalmology requires eight years of medical school, after which they are licensed to perform surgery. If you wanted to explore iridology, an alternative diagnostic approach to someone's health through the iris, people who may have specific training in it could be homeopaths, naturopaths, or possibly some chiropractors.

Teeth/Mouth: An oral and maxillofacial surgeon treats injury, disease, or defects to the hard and soft tissues of the face, jaws, and mouth. For general issues, see a dentist, and for alignment, an orthodontist. Surgery such as root canals or other issues in the interior of the tooth require an endodontist, which is a dentist with several more years of medical training. Interestingly, less than 3 percent of dentists are endodontists. They often are able to save diseased teeth, whereas standard dentistry cannot.

Cancer/Autoimmune: To diagnose cancer, an oncologist is the specialist to see. Oncology, surgery, and radiation therapy are the three venues of cancer treatment. If the issue is autoimmune-related, it might be best to see a rheumatologist, who treats rheumatic diseases like lupus, scleroderma, and rheumatoid arthritis.

Allergies: If it's allergies you need help with, an allergist or immunologist can diagnose and treat allergies. NAET (Nambudripad's Allergy Elimination Technique) through a naturopath also works with allergies.

Skin, Bone, Connective Tissue, and Organ Therapies

From here, we will discuss skin, bone, connective tissue, and what that entails as well as learn about each organ. I will pair body therapies with each group to help you get a better gauge on where to go if these areas are of issue.

Skin

We start with the largest organ in the body, the skin. When something is out of balance, many times it shows itself through the skin: skin rashes, bumps, color changes, patches of dryness, redness, changes in moles, and so on. Our skin must not only be taken care of, but we must always keep watch on it and look for any changes that might occur. Skin is one of the major places that our bodies use to communicate with us. Pay attention and take action when things change at the skin level. It always means something. Remember, nothing in the body works by itself, therefore if something is showing through your skin, there is always a message to be received. The more you ignore these things, the louder your body is going to have to speak in order to get through to you.

Detox and Body Cleansing

We all need to detox on a regular basis in the body, as well as the mind of things that surround us that do not serve our best purpose. To detox implies that you are ridding the body/mind/spirit of unwanted excess. You can detox through a multitude of avenues. You can detox your friends list, you can detox your way of thinking, or through the foods you eat or through body practices. You can detox your physical body by removing unwanted waste in the body. It's in the extracting of the unwanted where we can experience great comfort and pleasure and offer room for better things to build.

Body Scrub to Rid Dead Skin Cells

Taking care of the skin is extremely important as a daily habit. Body scrubs that help exfoliate the skin are a wonderful thing to do on a regular basis (weekly or biweekly; daily can nullify any benefit). Skin cells gather and die unevenly, therefore exfoliation is a wonderful way to slough off the parts that are no longer effective. You don't have to buy expensive exfoliators when it's easy to make something from your own kitchen; it's just as effective and you know exactly what is in it. Use coarse salt or sugar mixed with a carrier oil such as coconut, jojoba, grapeseed, apricot, avocado, or olive that can be used anywhere on the skin. You can put the mix in a bowl and then scoop it up with your fingers and rub it on the skin. It doesn't matter whether you rub up and down or in circles—go with your preference. After you've covered your body with the scrub, use a washcloth or simply rinse under the shower water to gently scrub off the mixture and reveal healthy, glowing skin. Some people also use coffee grounds to exfoliate, which is lovely because it gives the grounds another beneficial use.

Adding essential oils to a scrub mixture can be a delightful addition. It is advised to use high-quality, therapeutic-grade oils. Because you are using a carrier oil along with the essential oils, you don't have to be as cautious as you would if you were applying the essential oils directly on the skin. Invigorating scents like eucalyptus, rosemary, peppermint, and/or spearmint can help open the sinuses and lead to a happy, energized feeling while scrubbing. Oils like lavender, ylang-ylang, sweet orange, geranium, rose, and bergamot can lead to a softer, more relaxed, and calming energy when added to the mix. Grounding oils such as patchouli, sage, frankincense, and myrrh can bring about an earthy aroma and help you to feel balanced and aligned with the earth's energies. No matter which oil you choose, you don't need more than three to five drops of any essential oils to your bowl for the desired effect.

✽ PRACTICE: DETOX BATH

Doing simple things like taking a detox bath is something everyone can do to help their bodies get rid of heavy metals and heavy thoughts. I take a salt bath once a week and take a mustard bath at the change of the seasons to help clear the sinuses and encourage the release of toxins through the skin and urine with sweating and increased water intake.

My Go-To Detox Bath:

>1–2 cups Epsom salts
>
>1–2 cups sea salt

Optional:

>Aluminum-free baking soda, a pinch
>
>Essential oils, 3 to 5 drops

The salt pulls heavy metals from the body and calms sore muscles. I love to wash my face with the salt bath to cleanse and purify. Sit in the bath for around fifteen minutes or longer as hot as you can stand. Before I get in, I pour the salts in with really hot water. I fill it enough so that I can swirl it around and let the salt dissolve. Then I turn the water to a more comfortable temperature. There are tons of bath variations, but this detox bath is what I do on a weekly basis. Sometimes I only use the Epsom and not the sea salt. Then I just go for the full two cups or even dump in a large amount without measuring. As always, I trust my gut about what feels like the right amount.

I make it a point to take this detox bath after receiving a body treatment such as chiropractic, acupuncture, or massage; contrary to popular belief, the actual detoxification process does not happen in the bath—it's what you do *after* the bath that makes the difference. Salt or other bath therapies require a follow-up protocol: when you get out of the water, wrap yourself in a towel and climb in bed all the way under the covers (including the comforter) up to your chin with your arms tucked in. Allow your body to sweat out all the impurities the salts have pulled to the surface. After all, sweating through the pores is much more effective than just drinking a lot of water. Lie there for about ten minutes and let the sweat flush out of every pore in your body. Once you've sweat it out (you'll get a feeling of "I am done"), kick off those covers and drink some water. If you want to rinse off in the shower, go ahead—it's always a wise thing to do after a detox.

————————

If you need to detox but still haven't found the right avenue, maybe look for someone who does the ionic footbaths. Generally, chiropractors, naturopaths, colon hydrotherapists, and homeopaths have access to ionic footbaths, which can help detox heavy metals and other things from the body that need releasing. One friend of mine even experienced worms coming out of her feet in an ionic bath, but I've never personally experienced or seen that with my own foot baths or those of my clients.

Colon hydrotherapy can be very helpful in cleaning and detoxing the gut. Be sure to check with your doctor and/or hydrotherapist if you are currently dealing with a significant illness and make sure it's not a contraindication to your treatment. Colon hydrotherapy is a powerful way to release and start anew. While receiving a colonic, the therapist can tell you what is coming out and what it means. For example, bubbles may be yeast from excess sugar. It's amazing the things you can find out from the people who have spent their lives studying a specific area of healing! A colon hydrotherapist can likely tell you from what you release what you might be in need of for nutrient balancing. Just be open to what your body may need; if you haven't tried it before, do your research. As always, find someone that is highly qualified and fully credentialed to help you. Never be afraid to ask to see those credentials!

There are incredible mud or body wraps that help the skin release toxins as well. If you go to the spa, these can be fairly pricey … but if you have a school nearby, they can be very affordable. They may use a brush to apply the mixture, which is usually mud or clay-based but may also contain other minerals. It is applied over the body, and then you are wrapped up for the detox to trap in moisture. The wrapping in this little cocoon helps the body release. Thankfully, there are showers on location for you to rinse yourself off afterwards. The skin will be clean, purified, and you will feel calm and relaxed. It's a win-win treatment when you need one.

Looking Deeper into the Skin

When we are faced with a new challenge in our body, it is wise to look for the metaphor. If we break out in hives, pimples, or have eczema, often times we ask ourselves "What's gotten under my skin?" Always look at the metaphor as an option, because learning the right questions to ask yourself can offer insight when collecting information to formulate a plan of action. Don't get caught in the trap of missing the physical role the body plays in asking questions too. Asking the same questions of a new skin issue regarding the physical can include, "Have I made any changes in my diet?" "Is this occurring around the time of menstruation?" (Or, "When in the month is this happening?") "What changes have I made to my skin care regimen?" We must go down the full list looking into each of the aspects in full. Next is the emotional check-in with yourself. What are the changes that have been happening in your life at this time? Are you feeling depressed or anxious? Has there been a change in people or situations in your life recently? Is there added pressure in school or at work that is affecting you? These questions are all part of your overall body scan. You have to learn how to tap into the body in a different way by asking all possible questions to yourself. Once you can pinpoint the area that might have the most effect, you can figure out if you can work this out on your own or if you need to see somebody. If the latter, then you can decide which category of people to seek. You're not going to seek a psychologist or counselor (emotional) if you know that the area that has had the most change is something in your diet (physical). What if you had given up sugar or coffee or something significant in your diet just before the onset of skin irritations? Asking the right questions is paramount in finding the best answers.

It's common to refer to people as having thin and thick skin, and we don't necessarily mean the amount of subcutaneous fat that attaches to the layer of pinchable skin. If we perceive someone as being thick-skinned, it means they are able to take some of the rougher attitudes and criticisms thrown at them. Someone who has thin skin is perceived as being weak or overly sensitive.

The skin's tone and color matter as well. For example, a person who eats well and spends time in some sort of reflection or contemplation tends to have a glow to their skin. If I were to compare it to makeup, the skin would have a shiny finish. Habits such as excessive alcohol, smoking, or diet-related excess tend to flatten or matte the skin's appearance. The face takes on a duller appearance when nutrients are lost and can harden or even age faster when emotional health is out of balance. Many things show up on the skin, especially on your face, It's important to pay attention.

An Ayurvedic practitioner would look at your skin as part of determining your overall constitution. From your skin they can answer the questions concerning the diet that could bring you back into a proper alignment. The skin often is a large indicator of what might be out of balance. In looking at the skin's color or presentation, dull skin can signal a lack of certain nutrients.

I am a manual lymphatic drainage therapist also trained in something called combined decongestive therapy. I work with people after surgery, post cancer treatment, people with sluggish immune systems, acne, primary and secondary lymphedema, lipidema (fat disorder), and so on. The decongestive therapy aspect of my work is lymphatic massage, bandaging and compression, proper skin care, and proper exercise for the condition. The information that I have on skin is very unique. The method involves a series of movements in which the swelling caught underneath the skin is moved using an extremely gentle skin-stretching technique that guides the lymphatic fluid to a place in the body that has not been compromised where it can be properly digested and released via the urinary tract. It's incredible work—you can actually feel the liquid moving like sludge under the hands.

When doing standard regular massage therapy work that uses oils and creams, I feel for the skin texture in a totally different way. I can tell the difference in the feeling of the skin between someone who drinks more soda or alcohol than water. If a client smokes, the pores on the back open like a geyser when releasing toxins and buildup—I can actually smell the smoke releasing from the body. I've become intimately familiar with the skin on a whole different level, just like skin care practitioners such as estheticians and dermatologists, who have a long list of questions they run through when they do their work.

When the skin is pinched, the rate at which it returns to its original state can tell so much about its elasticity. For instance, if you have young, supple skin and pinch the back of the hand, it will quickly bounce back into its original place. As we age, it takes longer for the skin to go back to its original place when pinching the same area. Some people pinch this area and count how long it takes for the skin to return to normal as a way of associating our chronological age with our apparent age (add a zero after however many numbers it took to return to its original starting position; a count of four would indicate someone being forty in age according to that skin test). Notice in people's faces that their skin begins to age if they are lacking in nutrients such as amino fatty acids so necessary for glowing and radiant skin (this includes avocado and coconut oil, nuts, and fish such as wild-caught salmon). When I was first teaching aerobics, one of the trainers told me the most important thing I always needed to do before I taught a class was to wash my face. He stressed it was important not to sweat while wearing makeup. He said that everything gets into the cracks of the skin and ages us. The same is true for removing makeup before going to sleep at night.

Bone

Bones are considered a rigid organ of the body. They are also your primary source of support both physically and metaphysically. The bones are what makes up our skeletal system. Bones protect our vital organs and allow us to move about in our bodies. Otherwise, we'd be a sack of meat draped over what? Bone marrow deep in the center of our bones are where red and white blood cells are produced. Bones are what releases and stores both fat and minerals. Bones are serious business for a multitude of things.

When we think of osteoporosis, chances are we think of the older adult population who are more susceptible to breaking hips and bones. Osteoporosis is a disease where the bones become brittle and weak, such that even simple movements such as a strong cough can result in bone breakage. Sadly, osteoporosis is heavily prevalent among female athletes; girls who overtrain for sports or starve themselves through anorexic behaviors often have among the highest rates of osteoporosis. Smokers also have a high rate of this disease. The bones are naturally strong and supple unless someone is genetically predisposed for issues such as bone dysplasia, osteoarthritis, or due to lifestyle factors.

What are those lifestyle factors? Everything you do in your life affects how your body will carry you, and bones are no exception. Take note of any physical feelings in your bones *and* how you are feeling emotionally and spiritually. Are you getting the support you need? Do you feel as though your dreams, goals, and intentions are in alignment and are being carried out by you and those in your life? It's also important to check your vitamin levels and be sure that you are getting enough vitamin D and calcium, the foundations for strong and happy bones. Above all, there is no better source of vitamin D than what the body naturally absorbs from the sun. Be sure you are getting out into the sun, breathing in fresh air and giving yourself enough time in nature's embrace.

Osteopathy

Osteopathic medicine is a type of alternative practice that involves manual adjustments and physical manipulations to bones, muscle, and tissue. Osteopaths also perform myofascial release similar to craniosacral therapy. In fact, Dr. John Upledger, creator of Upledger Craniosacral Therapy, was an osteopathic physician. The level of understanding and appreciation for this incredible work varies around the world in different countries. In the United States, a person could either be a doctor of medicine (MD) or a doctor of osteopathic medicine (DO). Both MDs and DOs are fully licensed medical doctors. The course work is similar, but their approach to healing and function of the body vary greatly. A DO can perform surgery and prescribe medication as needed along with the practice of treating the whole body and erring on the side of healing through a whole-body approach.

Tissue

Have you ever heard the expression "the issues are in your tissues"? Do we even know what the word "tissues" refers to? Soft tissue in the body is practically everything—basically anything that isn't an organ or bone. The term can refer to tendons (connecting muscle to bone), ligaments (connecting bone to bone), fascia (a layer that covers everything, akin to panty hose), muscles (being the largest of the soft tissue), nerves, and even protein, fat, and blood vessels are considered part of the soft tissue, though not connective tissue. If it all sounds confusing, don't worry; we will delve into each topic deeper because all of them are extremely important to how we approach healing.

Blood/Plasma

Blood and plasma are vital to your overall health and well-being. Blood pumps the oxygen to your heart and supplies it to all your cells and tissues. It also pumps the carbon dioxide byproduct to the lungs so that it can be exhaled. And it *also* removes waste and is responsible for transporting hormones. Blood is the passageway that allows every organ in your body to do its job and is how cells are nourished and remain healthy. It carries life and life force. Red blood cells carry oxygen, white blood cells fight infections, platelets help stop bleeding due to injury, and plasma is how protein and other nutrients travel through your body.

In another sense, blood is family. If someone has committed horrible sins, we say that blood is on their hands. The common theme across the descriptions physical, metaphysical, and everything in between is that blood binds us. In Chinese Medicine, the blood and plasma are the carriers of memory throughout the body. It carries in it the genetic code passed down through the generations. It has its own wisdom and information within it. It is believed there is incredible power and sacredness of bleeding by menstruation (a time when a woman's energy is strongest and her intuition is highest). It is birth, creation, salvation, passion, life, and death.

By drawing blood, we can learn just about anything we need to know for diagnosis, birth charting, ancestry, genetic predispositions, and even what food/drink would be best for us to consume. A lack of blood can take life just as receiving blood can give life. If you want to truly tie something into your energy, put a little of your own blood on it. Blood has been used in ritual since the beginning of ritual itself. In old times, the most powerful sacrifices were often blood, although I would never suggest this practice! Blood is powerful, sacred, and mysterious. Eight different types of blood exist in the world, and I hope as you read this you already know your own blood type. If not, take the time to go find out what it is. Knowing your blood type can save a lot of time in crisis should you ever be in one. Blood is magic.

Muscle

My love affair with human anatomy, physiology, and bodywork centers around the muscles. Muscles are my jam; I have always loved them. Muscles by definition are bands of fibrous tissue that contract, lengthen, and produce movement. Muscles are associated with strength and power. According to my own research and beliefs, however, muscles store not just memory for movement but also emotions. The center of every muscle stores the experiences our bodies have endured throughout our lives. If a stimulus occurs that reminds the body of something painful, the body and the muscles know to flinch in response, even if that stimulus does not produce physical or emotional pain. Your muscles remember your life story and hang on tight to pain, just as pain can be stored in the mind, like a file cabinet of your ups and downs. The muscles also experienced the traumas and treasures of your life. Movements can reproduce bodily memories that were happy, healthy, and strong just as they can remember days of sadness and grief. The muscles have so much more wisdom than we realize. In my practice with clinical and neuromuscular massage therapy, I work with the muscles and have learned to develop the skill to listen to the muscles' messages. I find that when the muscles signal to my hands where they have physical pain, they also have emotional holds in the same space. Where we carry pain in our body tells a lot about our emotional attachments.

Treating the physical body through hands-on clinical massage therapy is something I relish. Addressing both the physical aspects as well as the potential emotional holding patterns within the muscles offers so much more potential for release and healing. To place my hands on the muscles and feel the pull from the body sets off a wildfire inside me!

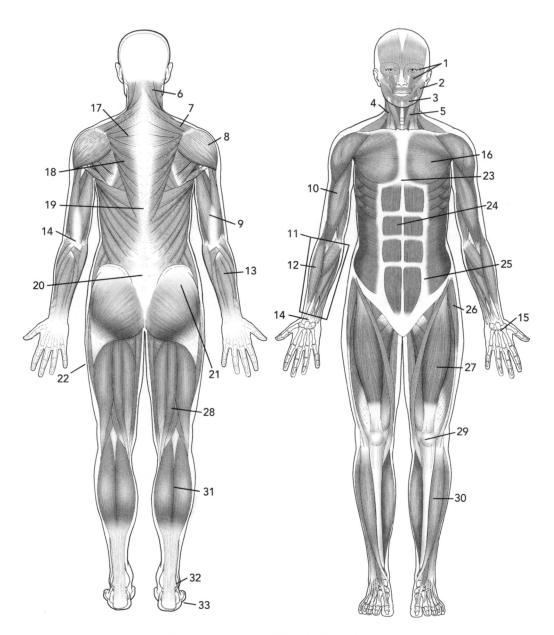

Figure 1: Emotional Muscle Chart Recap

Head/Neck

1. Facial expressions: cheeks—smile/frown, eyes—true happiness or sadness
2. Jaws: tension and replaying of socially painful situations
3. Chin: muscles of sadness
4. Lateral neck muscles: flexibility and awareness of your surroundings
5. Anterior neck muscles: secret keepers of pain and trauma
6. Back of the neck: stress generally caused from outside influences

Shoulders

7. Tops of shoulders: weight of the world, too much stress, requiring excessive control
8. Side of shoulders/deltoids: also carrying excess baggage and embracing change

Arms

9. Triceps: pushing away, repel something
10. Biceps: embracing, acceptance

Forearms

11. Whole forearms relate to the throat chakra, speaking up and being heard
12. Extensors (tops of the forearms) repel, push away
13. Flexors (bottom palm side of the forearms) pull in, accept, bring to
14. Wrists and elbows: ability to redirect
15. Hands: the maps same as feet. Helps assimilate information and feedback.

Chest

16. Brings in love, or repels too much emotion. Correlates to the heart chakra.

Back

17. Upper back/trapezius same as tops of the shoulders—too much stress, need to be in control, weight of the world
18. Shoulder blades area: betrayal being stabbed in the back
19. Middle center of the back: support muscles, strength in alignment with choices and movement
20. Lower back: fear of financial difficulties, fear of moving forward, loss

Glutes (buttocks)

21. Aggravation and suppression
22. IT band (begins in center of glutes but runs down the outside of the leg) confidence, and safety make this muscle work well

Abdomen/Psoas

23. Diaphragm: confidence and trust
24. Abdominal wall: protection over vital organs and decisions within the body
25. Psoas: vulnerable, secret keeper

Legs

26. Hips: gatherers of information/decision making
27. Quads: protection, strength in movement, supports forward motion
28. Hamstrings: support muscles and offers follow through in movement and decisions
29. Knees: making decisions, or feeling stuck. Forward motion keeps knees healthy.
30. Anterior Tibialis (shins): follow through on moving in a forward direction
31. Calves: is your heart in it?
32. Ankles: the sweetness in life, are you allowing time for pleasure?
33. Feet: the maps. They feel, assimilate information and form decisions

Anatomy, origin, insertion, structure, function, and fiber direction within the muscles themselves are exciting, so it's amazing to understand and work my way through each area of the body. I love to shake up and realign a client's body in a way that makes them feel in tune and back in balance. If you need to address your muscle body and don't know where to begin, check the final section of the book for a list of modalities and specialties for bodywork.

Massage

Massage therapy is a series of manual manipulations of the body's soft tissues (muscles, connective tissues, tendons, ligaments) done with the intention to enhance a person's health and wellness. Massage therapy can be a highly specialized healing practice depending on who you go to for such work. Being that my training is through clinical and neuromuscular massage therapy with an advanced study of lymphatic drainage, massage therapy to me is one of the greatest untapped treasures in all of the world for authentic healing applications. There are so many incredible massage styles and healing practices around the world. Because massage is a hands-on healing practice where we are trained to treat almost the entire body, some people take advantage of this sacred practice and use it as a front to behave badly. This gives massage a bad rap when in truth, the healing treasures behind the majority of this hands-on practice are powerful beyond simple description. Massage practices such as Tui Na of Chinese Medicine is a highly sought-after medical massage practice that takes a minimum of five years to learn. Practices like Lomi Lomi out of Hawaii and Ayurvedic massage with oils blended according to your dosha practiced in India are also increasing in popularity in the West. Shiatsu, practiced in Japan, uses various pressure techniques, and Thai massage from Thailand stretches the body and lengthens the muscle. Lymphatic drainage is used primarily for post-surgery, illness and recovery, post-cancer, and chronic swelling conditions such as lymphedema and lipidema. Pre- and post-natal massage require extensive training especially if you go down the path of the Arvigo training for working with the expectant mother and beyond. There is massage work you would find in a spa such as Swedish, deep tissue, body wraps, aromatherapy massage, hot stone massage, and so on. There are also specialties you might find in a spa such as a Vichy shower where the person lies under the water that sprays down like a massage while a massage therapist adds the work in alongside the shower. There is also Ashiatsu, where there are bars on the ceiling as they work on you through their feet. Some places offer a water massage called Watsu where the practitioner will glide you through the water for lengthening the muscles and relaxing the body. There are also highly clinical massage practices that a person would go to for injury prevention and treatment such as myofascial release, orthopedic massage, myoskeletal alignment, clinical massage, neuromuscular massage therapy, sports massage, trigger point therapy, Rolfing, and structural integration. There are also stretching practice such as PNF (proprioceptive, neuromuscular facilitation), ART (active release therapy), Thai massage, and Thai Yoga Therapy. There are so many beautiful styles to choose from, and each is incredible if you find a wonderful and skilled therapist.

Fascia

Fascia is connective tissue, but not all connective tissue is fascia (confusing, I know). Fascia is the connective tissue that holds together, separates, *or* binds tissues of the body, and it covers both muscles and organs—my teacher described it as the body's panty hose. Fascia is everywhere in the body and exists in different densities in different places. Here's a simple analogy to help you understand fascia: imagine you are wearing a tight-fitting shirt, and you tug on one corner of the shirt. When you do this, you notice that the whole shirt pulls down as a reaction to the bottom corner being pulled. That is how fascia works in and around our muscles and organs. If the fascia has a restriction pattern, the whole body will be affected and follow a line outward from that restriction point.

Sometimes when we assume a body problem is just a tight muscle, it could easily be a restriction in the fascia instead. To restore the range of motion, it will be necessary to unwind the restriction. Fascia restrictions can wreak havoc on the physical, emotional, and energetic bodies, and it's amazing what can happen when these restrictions are released. Working with the fascia in the area of the brain and spinal cord can release not just the fascial restrictions but also restrictions in the blood and cerebral spinal fluids that transport vital nutrients to the brain. Upledger Craniosacral Therapy works to help alleviate restrictions in the body, especially in the bones and membrane layers surrounding the brain and spinal cord. Through this work therapists are able to alleviate symptoms of several disorders within the brain such as autism spectrum symptoms, sensory processing disorders, ADD/ADHD, and concussions or other trauma to the brain, among other things. It is through this work that my child was able to become verbal and recover from her autism diagnosis. Removing these types of restrictions are the foundation for

Upledger Craniosacral Therapy. When it comes to therapies that work with the fascia such as craniosacral therapy, myofascial release, acupuncture, acupressure, and EFT (emotional freedom technique), all are power players in healing because what they do is unwind the fascia and remove the restriction patterns that have been holding you back. Dry needling is another practice in which many have found great relief from pain through unwinding the fascia and clearing the lactic acid within the muscles. Remember, there is no place where the fascia doesn't run within the body. Fascia work is subtle but the results are powerful.

Nerves

Nerves are bundles of fibers that transmit impulses of sensation by way of the brain and spinal cord through the muscles and organs. Nerves run through the muscles and all soft tissue of the body and serve as the body's information superhighway. The nervous system is the foundation for everything to work within our bodies. It's the feedback station for literally everything that happens. In a nutshell, it's the internet for our body's communication.

Chiropractic

Chiropractic is a form of alternative medicine that works with the spine and musculoskeletal system. If you visit a chiropractor, you will likely receive a manual adjustment of the neck and spine. This adjustment helps balance the central nervous system (brain and spinal cord) and is a kind of spinal manipulation that improves the body's function and movement. It is done either with the hands or a small instrument to apply controlled force to a spinal joint. Most people seek adjustments to ease neck, back, head, and ear pains.

Chiropractors do not meet Western medicine requirements to be considered a person's primary care provider, although many people prefer to visit their chiropractor in place of a family care doctor due to the extensive studies and whole body healing approach that many chiropractors take. When it comes to finding the best chiropractor for you, due diligence is a must—there are so many out there, and some are masterful body wizards who can help you achieve incredible and miraculous results. There are also many out there who ask you to visit them several times a week, as if they are only after your money. The Mayo Clinic reports that most people attain "maximum improvement in six to ten visits."[7] Generally, the chiropractor will take X-rays of your spine before beginning the course of treatment.

Chiropractic offers a large platform for many additional treatment modalities and take a whole-body approach to healing, but they are not licensed to prescribe medications. I have met some of the most incredibly trained body healers in the world who were chiropractors by trade. Many practice herbology, naturopathy, diet therapy, hyperbaric chamber therapy, Bach Flower remedies, chelation therapy (for heavy metals), vitamin drips for healing from major diseases such as cancer, testing of hair for heavy metals, and much more. Your job is to find the one who has the most knowledge that suits your needs.

Muscle-Fascia-Nerves Action

Here is where the muscle body, the fascia, and the nerve bundles all come together, but each with their own distinct energy. The muscles store emotions and memory and then are felt and experienced through the nerve tracks that carry the sensations to the brain for feedback response. Fascia moves energy and memory along its own matrix, and it also experiences emotions and memories which are moved differently than the muscles. Memories are stored deep in the muscles, felt by the nerves and then moved and released by way of the fascia. Muscles are held in place and shaped by fascia. Fascia surrounds every muscle fiber in the body, but they are not the same things physically, energetically, or emotionally. Too many times we incorrectly lump them together into one group doing the same thing.

Fascia contains both touch receptors and nerve endings that affect the dynamics of how we perceive pain. The nerve endings are part of the central nervous system, and it is through the nerves that we feel physical pain. When muscles and fascia run through nerve plexus areas (areas of higher concentration of nerve bundles) this can signal a more vulnerable area of the body in terms of both pain receptors and emotional responses. The iliopsoas muscle, for example, located in the area outside and more superficial to the reproductive organs, is the body's primary hip flexor. The muscle originates in the spine and crosses the front of the body. This muscle also crosses through the lumbar plexus of the spine, a highly energized area for feeling and experiencing vulnerable emotions. Its

7. Mayo Clinic, "Chiropractic adjustment." https://www.mayoclinic.org/tests-procedures/chiropractic-adjustment /about/pac-20393513.

location and connection constitute one reason the iliopsoas is one of the most emotionally charged muscles in our bodies.

Naturopathy

The study of naturopathy is a system of beliefs that disease can be reversed or prevented without the use of drugs and pharmaceutical medications. Believers report that techniques such as exercise, massage therapy, healing touch, meditation, and diet can alter a person's health in the most significant ways. Under a naturopath, there are many specialties one would practice and finding someone who works in the realm of what you are looking for is the key. My family sees our naturopath for a treatment called NAET (Nambudripad's Allergy Elimination Technique), which is specific work that helps us get over food and other bodily sensitivies. This treatment worked to help me overcome the final experiences of my anxiety, and it's worked with my children for skin conditions, behaviors, emotions, and foods. Other things my naturopath works with are the Bach Flower remedies and other natural treatments. Many naturopaths use infrared saunas, ionic footbaths, and hyperbaric chambers, among other things, to help many imbalances.

Kinesiotesting

Applied Kinesiology, or kinesiotesting is a way to communicate with the body through the muscles, sometimes referred to as muscle testing. It is a direct path to communication with the body to measure how it responds to something through the muscles. When I spoke with Dr. Tom Dill, he explained that "the body communicates in a binary code. Yes or no. Good or bad. The two energies feel very different. Good feels very different than bad. It's one or the other; there aren't shades of gray." Kinesiotesting is an easy shortcut to find out if something resonates with your body or it doesn't. To put it bluntly, he cuts through the bullshit and gets right to it: when he tests any issue, he tests for three things: (1) structure—is it something in the patient's physical structure? (2) environmental—is it something in the home, workplace, or any other place in life? (3) emotional—is it the way a patient responds to something or the way they feel about it? Once he determines from which area the issue is coming, he then proceeds to treat for it according to that avenue of expression. Personally, these treatments have yielded far more powerful and longer-lasting results than trying to get my mind to shift around the ideas and concepts.

It is important to note that when a kinesiologist is asking your body questions, they are not spoken aloud. That is, I do not know what answers my body gives to him. For example, he asks me to hold my arm out straight and resist. Sometimes I can hold a hundred pounds and my arm will stay firm, and other times I couldn't hold it up if I was begged to. It's important that the conscious mind does not interfere with the testing process, which is why nothing is asked verbally. It's a wonderful tool to use for children because they aren't required to discuss emotions that they do not yet understand how to articulate.

There are ways in which a person can kinesiotest themselves. Some people hold their thumb and ring finger together and try not to separate them as they ask questions, commonly referred to as the O ring test. For example, if they are testing a particular product to see if the body would react positively to it, they may hold the bottle against their chest and connect their thumb and ring finger of the arm that is holding the product. With the other hand, they try to separate the fingers by pulling them apart to see if it reacts strong or weak, where "strong" means that the fingers easily stay together and "weak" means they are easily separated. You must be very clear with yourself when testing with what you believe "strong" and "weak" mean for any given answer, because consistency is key. The other easy way to test anything is called the tip test: stand with your feet shoulder-width apart and not locked. Take whatever product you are testing to see if it's strong or weak/ good or bad for you. Whatever you are testing put it to your chest and close your eyes. Your body will either move forward or backward slightly. It's a very quick response though not very obvious in movement. If you tip forward, it means the response is strong and your body is moving toward it. If your body tips backward, it is repelled by it. If nothing happens and you remain still, it likely means your body is indifferent to the product. You might try this practice at the grocery store with two identical products made by different manufacturers; tip test one and then the other to see if one is better or both are fine.

Essential Oils/Aromatherapy

Essential oils are all the rage these days, and for good reason—they have incredible healing properties that help treat emotions as well as enhance or balance physical issues. That said, quite a few are harmful when applied directly to the skin (such as eucalyptus and bergamot), so it is recommended to see an herbalist who has studied essential oils and knows how to make blends specific to your needs. Essential oils can be used for a great many reasons but should *not* be a substitute for medical practices. Too many people regard them as completely safe, even encouraging ingesting the oils (something I don't recommend)!

Essential oils are powerful because they are highly concentrated and thus need to be treated with respect and awareness. When choosing them, always select the highest, cleanest grade possible. Learning to mix your oils with a carrier oil such as jojoba, olive oil, grapeseed oil, avocado oil, or apricot kernel oil is an important part of using essential oils as aromatherapy and if you are considering applying them to the skin. Be careful, however, as there are many oils that are dangerous to your pets, especially when used through the diffuser. Some examples are: tea tree, eucalyptus, sweet birch, citrus, cinnamon, pennyroyal, ylang-ylang, peppermint, wintergreen, tea tree, lavender, oregano, clove, thyme, juniper anise, and yarrow. As well, all alliums (garlic, onions, chive, etc.) are harmful for dogs.[8]

CBD Products

There is so much information about CBD (cannabidiol) oils out there that it can be hard to find what type of product to choose and how it would help. Some people have reported incredible results when adding CBD oil to their daily regimen to address issues of inflammation, pain, anxiety, and sensory issues, as well as a reduction of the amount, duration, and intensity of seizures. Cannabidiol is a derivative of the hemp plant but does not contain (or contains only trace amounts less than a percent) of the element THC, which is responsible for the "high" conventionally associated with marijuana. CBD is not a drug; it is legal and can be a very safe alternative to many prescription medications. Think of CBD as a plant-based remedy that has done wonders in the world of alternative medicine (or traditional medicine, to be more accurate). CBD can be found in products that can be ingested, applied to the skin, or inhaled through a vaporizer. As with most plants, organic is always best. Do plenty of research before making any choice, and keep in mind that you will likely not see the results or benefits you are looking for if the product is of poor quality. Learn your product—where it is farmed, harvested, handled, and manufactured.

Herbal Remedies

Using herbs for healing is a practice as old as time itself. Ancient medicine men and women gathered plants from the forest to make remedies that were sacred, powerful, and healing. You can do the same when you find the right products or consult an herbalist to

---

8. Shannon Casey, "Essential Oils and Animals: Which Essential Oils Are Toxic to Pets?" Michelson Found Animals. https://www.foundanimals.org/essential-oils-toxic-pets.

address specific conditions. Herbs are widely available these days but are most often found in natural food stores, and it's common to find Ayurvedic practitioners, Chinese Medicine practitioners, herbalists, naturopaths, and homeopaths, blending raw herbs to address specific health concerns. The practitioner may make a tea out of their combination of herbs either in their whole form or ground into a powder. Or they could sell pills from trusted sources that are already bottled and at the ready. As with CBD, it's best to find organically grown herbs or ones that were grown without the use of pesticides or harmful chemicals. When choosing herbal remedies, again be sure to do proper research and see someone you trust to guide your way.

Homeopathy

The principle of homeopathic medicine (considered a holistic practice of medicine) is based on the idea that what can cause something can also cure it; the same compound transmuted into different energy, or "like cures like." For example: arsenic is poison. However, take that original arsenic and dilute it thousands of times. Through a process known as succession, a person hits the compound many times in a way that allows the energy of the substance to permeate the biologically and energetically diluted version of the original. Now in liquid form, they pour it over very small bead-like sugar pills that soak in the new compound. Many times, homeopathic medicine is administered in these small pills. A person places the pills under the tongue to let them dissolve, ideally pouring it directly into the mouth without an energy transfer from the hands. This transformed version of the original can now cure whereas the concentrated amount would kill. When we tap into the body and pull out the emotions from the tissues through the combination of physical and energy work, that same emotion that caused the illness can now be used in a way that liberates the illness. The body can reprogram and allow itself to use that same energy behind the original source to heal itself completely. The idea that like cures like is also fundamental to energy healing with human touch or even the use of intention. It offers encouragement behind the idea that the body is able to recover itself. We must find the right combination to adjust what caused the trauma and grief and turn it into liberation.

In the United States, homeopathic medicine is not regarded as it is in European countries and other places around the world. Because there are so few practitioners here in the states, many times the appointments are done over video call with the homeopathic physician and then they create their formulas based on your discussion. They need to be able to see you, however; generally they won't take audio-only appointments. This type of medicine is very detailed and requires many years of diligent study.

Bach Flower Remedies

A tip for getting a handle on stress when it comes up is to use natural homeopathic flower essences such as Bach Flower *Rescue Remedy* to calm the nervous system (I always keep it handy in my purse). You can find them in any health food store. All you do is put a few drops (the bottle says up to four) under the tongue and in just a few minutes you will find that your breath, your thoughts, and your body will all be calm. There are thirty-eight Bach Flower remedies that address a variety of issues. If you see a practitioner who knows how to blend certain remedies into something specific to your needs, it can serve as a wonderful way to cut through the layers of emotions to help you heal.

Bach Flower essences do not work on illness but treat emotions instead. However, I offer this in the physical section because they treat the emotions through the flower remedies, which are physical substances. Using a Bach Flower remedy is like cutting directly through an onion of emotions rather than peeling it layer by layer. As with other natural healing modalities, it is subtle in its approach and quite powerful in its response. Bach Flower remedies cast out emotions such as hate, worry, fears, indecision, and other negative emotions that leave the emotional body unbalanced. There are blends specifically for pets, babies, children, expecting mothers, and everyone in between.

Organs

An organ is a specific part of the body that serves a vital function in keeping us alive. There are five vital organs that ensure life: heart, liver, kidneys, lungs, and brain. Other organs include the bladder, small and large intestines, pancreas, spleen, gallbladder, colon, and stomach. In truth, it is believed that there are up to seventy-nine organs in our bodies, though there is controversy about what constitutes an organ. I have listed what I consider to be the most noteworthy.

According to Chinese Medicine each organ corresponds to its own emotion, as well as peak time and low times for energy and strength. Each organ also has a flavor profile that pairs with each organ's physical responsibility. It can be easy when you know the emotions that pair to the organ to get lost in assuming that this is the only emotion this area of the body might offer for you to experience. For this reason, I will offer a meditation with

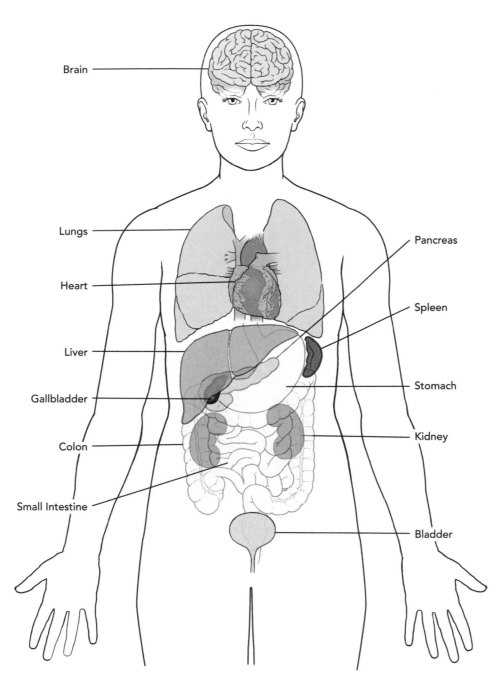

Figure 2: The Body's Organs

the organs and not list the emotional pair because I want you to feel for yourself without being influenced what yours might hold. Not everything you feel is charted somewhere, nor does it mean you are wrong and someone else is right (this includes my work with muscles and emotions as well). Go through your body, feel the area, and get to know each organ. Try to feel the emotions that you might experience in this journey. I'm going to offer the organ information by way of the following meditation train station.

⌘ Practice: Hands-on Organ Feeling and Listening Stations

To listen to this meditation, go to my website, emilyafrancisbooks.com, and click on the CDs tab. I've uploaded a free audio track of this meditation if you prefer to listen to the meditation in place of reading it.

Make sure you have already used the rest room before beginning this exercise. Lie down comfortably in a place that you can relax for however long this might take. Remove distractions such as lights, your phone, TV, and uncomfortable clothing.

Close your eyes and slow your breathing. With each deep breath in and out, clear away mental distractions. Allow your breathing to guide the way. Begin by placing your hands at your lower abdomen just above the pubic bone to the bladder. The word is *release.* Make sure both palms of the hands lie flat against the area side by side allowing energy to reveal itself to you. Clear your internal space and listen. Are any thoughts, messages, or feelings coming to you now? Check in with the energy in this area. Try to blend into the rhythm of the blood and urine flow. Does it feel healthy, vibrant, fluid without disruption?

Move the hands up to cover the navel. Circling the area around the navel just beneath it is the small intestine. Moving wider around the small intestine is the large intestine. Feel this area, listen to its messages. What does it have to share with you? Above the intestines and slightly situated to the left side and slightly higher is the stomach. Behind the stomach is the pancreas. The word for the small intestine, large intestine, stomach, and pancreas is *digestion.* Listen to any gurgles and try to hear or feel any messages that might come through. Rest and digest live in this area. Tap into it and feel its energy.

Move your hands slightly left from the stomach and a little bit up toward the chest to feel for your spleen. Think of your spleen as your cleaning station for the blood. The spleen is important to your body's immune system. It recycles the old red blood cells and stores the white blood cells and platelets. It is little but it is fierce. The word is *recycle*. Move your hands to the right side just below the right rib cage to find the liver and just below the liver, the gallbladder. The liver can be thought of as your superstation of creation. It helps with a zillion things in the body. The word is *metabolic*. There is a strong emotional charge within the liver. The gallbladder sits just below the liver and they are often clumped as one because they work so tightly together. The gallbladder is more of a holding station. The word is *storage*. It is shaped like a little pear tucked away under the liver.

What are the emotions that sit underneath your hands at each stop? Are you receiving any messages from the body without preconceived notions? Bring your hands behind you just below the rib cage on both sides of the back to connect with the kidneys. The word is *filter*. Kidneys remove waste from the blood which then turns into urine to exit the body. Sitting above the kidneys are the adrenal glands and they are shaped like a little bell. Adrenal glands are home to adrenaline, where the fight-or-flight reaction comes to life (think of adrenal glands as little warnings bells that ring when we get frightened). The word is *hormone*. Feel this area and the messages it may be bringing to you.

Bring your hands back to the front to the rib cage over the lungs on each side. One hand on each lung. Feel the breath, feel the air fill and expand, then leave and contract. The word is *respiration*. Listen deeply to the sounds of your lungs, feel the energy that lives inside this area. Ask it questions, check in with it. What are you feeling as you mold the energy of your hands into the lungs as they move?

Take your left palm and place it to the upper middle of the chest and slightly left to cover the heart. Place your right palm on top of your left palm to double up on heart space energy. The word is *pump*. Take it in. Give and receive the love in this space. Feel the blood pumping. Recognize the cardiac muscle movement that sits below your hands. Connect into its rhythm. Pumping the blood through the entire body, keeping you alive and well. Ask it questions and listen for the answers. Answers can come in tiny imprints into your mind. Words, sounds, or feelings can be communicated. Make sure that you not only ask for messages, but you offer it your love and gratitude for pumping every single moment of every single day of your life. Stay in this space as long as you need to before moving your hands.

Coming up to the head and tapping into your brain. Place both hands on your head covering as much surface area as you are able. Keep your eyes closed, relax the eyebrows and forehead. Try to connect and communicate with the motherboard of your body. The word is *control*. The brain is the whole body's distribution center. Feel all the synapses and movement happening within your brain in this moment. Do you feel any restrictions, bumps, or holding patterns? Talk with your brain directly. Listen to its messages.

Notice if your hands stop anywhere and what is being offered to you from within. Recognize and appreciate each vital organ that works without stopping throughout every moment of your life. Give thanks as your hands glide along each area of your body. Feel the energy of your entire body beneath your hands. Breathe deeply into this space. Feel the unity within your body. Give thanks.

To come out, keep your eyes closed until the end. Continue to breathe slow and deep and keep your eyes closed. Become aware of the air on your skin. Slowly wiggle your fingers and your toes. Bring your attention to the physical body and the outside world around you. Bring yourself back to the physical world slowly and with intention. When you are ready, slowly open your eyes and return to your day.

Chapter 5
The Physical Experience

Your physical body is the house in which your soul lives out this incarnation. But it's so much more than that. Isn't it mind blowing that while we do technically live out this one single incarnation in our current body, our DNA strands and cellular memory carry information and stored trauma passed down beyond this one life from generation to generation? Studies have now found that the DNA of Holocaust survivors pass down the trauma among later generations.[9] (And it's not just Holocaust survivors who are passing down information through the genetic codes. Studies have also shown that cellular trauma and memory through the ancestral line can affect how we react to similar stimulus in this life.[10])

Everything we experience comes through our bodies, and the physical body is the connection piece through which life on earth is experienced. We touch, feel, taste, suffer, delight, move, sleep, eat, use the bathroom, have sex. Every single thing we experience in the earth's cycle is experienced through our bodies. We do not understand life without our bodies once we arrive in it, and everything we experience with our basic five senses is felt through our physical self. Touch, taste, smell, sight, and sound as well as the elements earth, fire, air, water, metal, wood, and space (this is combination of elements taken from

9. Nagy A. Youssef, Laura Lockwood, Shaoyong Su, Guang Hao, Bart P. F. Rutten, "The Effects of Trauma, with or without PTSD, on the Transgenerational DNA Methylation Alterations in Human Offsprings," *Brain Sciences* 8, May 8, 2018. DOI: 10.3390/brainsci8050083.

10. Aaron Kase, "Science Is Proving Some Memories Are Passed Down From Our Ancestors" Reset.me. February 20, 2015. http://reset.me/story/science-proving-memories-passed-ancestors.

Chinese and Vedic and blended together because they all cover a defined term of elements) all affect our lives. The sacred breath is experienced through our physical self and then materializes its goodness throughout all of our body layers.

The Earth and All Her Glory

Walking outside and feeling the earth's natural offerings is a wonderful way to get in tune with your body in the physical plane. These natural wonders are some of the most blissful and enchanting sources for inspiration, good health, release, and rejuvenation. Everything in nature is an offering for us humans to protect, use, and enjoy. Enjoy the elements of wood as trees; water from lakes, rivers, and oceans; grass and dirt from the earth herself. Smelling the smells of nature, listening to the sounds of the birds and other creatures that sing her chorus. Take time when you are able to reach out and touch those trees and connect into the roots to ground yourself. Never pass on the chance to marvel at Mother Nature's offerings to us. They are sacred gifts and tools that we can use each and every day for our healing, recovery, and contemplation.

According to research in the *Journal of Environmental and Public Health*: "Emerging scientific research has revealed a surprisingly positive and overlooked environmental factor on health. Direct physical contact with the vast supply of electrons on the surface of the Earth. Modern lifestyle separates humans from such contact. The research suggests that this disconnect may be a major contributor to physiological dysfunction and unwellness." It goes on to say, "Reconnection with the Earth's electrons has been found to promote intriguing physiological changes and subjective reports of well-being. Earthing (or grounding) refers to the discovery of benefits including better sleep and reduced pain—from walking barefoot outside or sitting, working, or sleeping indoors connected to conductive systems that transfer Earth's electrons from the ground into the body." The study goes on to suggest that fifteen minutes a day barefoot in the grass can help realign our energy frequency and lead to more vibrant health. The authors refer to it as a source of "electric nutrition" for the body.[11]

---

11. Gaetan Chevalier, Stephen T. Sinatra, James L. Oschman, Karol Sokal, Pawel Sokal, "Earthing: Health Implications of Reconnecting the Human Body to the Earth's Surface Electrons," *Journal of Environmental and Public Health.* January 12, 2012. DOI: 10.1155/2012/291541.

Moving Meditation: Earthing

Earthing can be done anywhere natural for any amount of time. It's a wonderful work break and is even more beneficial when used as an intentional meditation or centering practice. Whether it's for one minute or sixty minutes, do this as often as you possibly can for best results. This practice should be done outside, preferably in the grass or dirt—no sidewalks or concrete. Take your shoes off and begin to walk barefoot. Walk all around the grass, avoiding stepping on the flowers. Notice if the grass flattens as you walk, and if so, lighten your steps. Walk to feel the grass beneath your feet. Take in the earth energy and bring the energy from the ground up into your body through your feet. Lift your palms facing up and bring your arms out to each side. Feel the air on the hands, open the palms upward to the sky. Feel the grass at your feet and your connection between the heavens, the earth, and the air all around you. Lift your head up and feel the sun shine on your face. If you do this at night, feel the moonlight dance on your skin. Allow the elements that are all unspoiled parts of the earth, and bring their elemental energy into you. Now as you continue to move and walk, breathe through the soles of your feet. Breathe through your entire body and focus on the arches of your feet. Pull not just the earth energy up through that space, but now breathe into that space all the way up and out through the nose. Inhale through the feet. Exhale through the nose or mouth. Inhale, bring in the earth through your body, cleaning out all avenues that might be blocked in your physical body. Allow the elements to cleanse the body—air, earth, water, sun, moon. It's all elemental earth energy and is so much more healing and powerful than we think. Take it in through your feet and breathe in from the feet all the way up and out. Slow the pace and stand still. Keep your head facing up, palms facing up, feet planted firmly down, and toes spread out and gripping the ground beneath. Close your eyes and take in a few more breaths from your feet and through your body. Exhale deeply with a sigh through your mouth: Ahhh-hhh. "Ah" is the natural sound for release. It signals to our body and your mind to let go and surrender. Allow. Bring in. Find the balance. Connect and ground yourself into the earth. You are truly in your physical body in this moment experiencing the earth's energy. Give thanks before you move on into the rest of your day or evening.

Intentional Breathing

The breath of life comes from outside of your body as oxygen, and leaves your body by way of carbon dioxide. The inhaling of oxygen initiates all mechanisms of the internal body. Oxygen is the gift of the trees. To enhance your experience of deep breathing, it is advised to practice in the woods near as many trees as you can find, or sit near a single tree around your house. Next time you look at the trees around you, be sure to take an extra special deep breath and give gratitude to the trees that nourish your lungs.

In the tradition of yoga, the practice of breathing with intention is called Pranayama—the "breath of life." Where there is breath, there is always hope. There are many ways of practicing breathing; whatever way you choose likely will lead to a calming and centering of the mind and body and an invigorating lift to the blood, plasma, bones, and marrow. It will bring a lift to every other tissue and organism in your body. In Taoist philosophy, it is believed that we are born with a certain number of breaths and how we choose to use them—long or short—will determine the length of our life. When we are unhealthy, stressful, angry, sad, or short-tempered, the breath tends to be short, shallow, and high in the chest. A person who is rested, healthy, has a lighter mental disposition or who practices calming, restorative exercises (such as yoga, tai chi, qi gong, martial arts, meditation, and so on) tends to breathe from a lower area of the body. The breath is soft, silent, and the length of each breath is naturally longer. The more stress you are under, the louder the breath becomes, especially while sleeping. As far as lung capacity is related to how much oxygen we take in, 80 percent comes from the diaphragm, 10 percent from the chest/sternum, and the other 10 percent from the clavicle/collar bone. When we are anxious, angry, or emotional, we tend to only get 10 to 20 percent of our maximum capacity into the lungs because we are only breathing from the chest up, not from below the rib cage at the diaphragm.

Above every breathing practice I could explain is one important tip that gets overlooked way too often. When told to "take a deep breath," people tend to inhale deeply like they are about to put their face under water. What needs to happen instead is that the deep breath is first expelled from the body as an exhalation. Breathe everything out of your lungs first. Empty them so that when you take that deep breath in, there is room for the fresh air to enter. Do not create or exacerbate the potentially stressful condition you might already be under by forcing air into lungs that aren't empty. Professional swimmers have this trick down pat, but the rest of us somehow missed this very incredible piece of the breathing puzzle! If you don't believe me, watch a swimmer before a race starts. They get in the water and do a series of forced exhales before they take the vital starting breath that helps them subsist on the smaller breaths that get them across the pool.

Two breathing practices are offered here that are highly effective and super easy to follow. Please note that to increase the effectiveness of any breathing practice, try to bring the shoulder blades toward each other in the upper back to quickly open up the diaphragm, chest, and clavicle without effort or strain.

✖ PRACTICE: INTENTIONAL BREATHING 1

The easiest and most effective practice for coming into center, calming the mind, and energizing the body by way of oxygenating the blood is through this one simple set of breathing practice:

- Exhale for a count of four: 1, 2, 3, 4 Hold the breath for four: 1, 2, 3, 4.
- Inhale for a count of four: 1, 2, 3, 4 Hold the breath for four: 1, 2, 3, 4.
- Exhale and repeat.
- Exhale first, hold it there with the breath let out. Breathe in slowly and hold that breath. Then again exhale and hold it once you've released the breath. If you want to increase this practice you would do everything the same except that you would change the exhale count to eight but everything else is still a 4 count. It looks like this:
- Exhale for 1, 2, 3, 4, 5, 6, 7, 8 and hold 1, 2, 3, 4, inhale 1, 2, 3, 4 and hold 1, 2, 3, 4
- Exhale 1, 2, 3, 4, 5, 6, 7, 8 and hold 1, 2, 3, 4 repeat at least 4 full rounds.

✖ PRACTICE: INTENTIONAL BREATHING 2

This practice is specifically for times when you are feeling overwhelmed and need the breath to be focused; think of it as pressing the reset button of your mind and body. Take a drinking straw. Holding the straw with one hand, wrap your lips tightly around one end and exhale first through the straw and then inhale through the nose. With each exhale through the straw, be a little more forceful—really try to empty out your lungs through this tiny hole. Keep the straw in your mouth, and continue to inhale through your nose, exhale through the straw. Continue for at least ten breaths to get the body to reset itself and clear the clutter from your mind.

Touch

Touch is one of the Universe's most powerful healers. Many people report feeling better after physical contact that is loving, comforting, kind, nourishing, or nurturing. A simple hug, offered hand, or physical body treatment such as massage can work wonders. I consider touch without expectation of reciprocation to be part of the concept of unconditional love, and it does not have to be only physical acts of intimacy. It's a passing of love. What you do with it is entirely up to you. You don't have to give anything back, but you might want to pass it on. Or you might just want to sit with it and keep it. The gift is in the ability to accept. Touch without expectation is so powerful and so loving; my wish for everyone is to receive it on a regular basis. Whether from a significant other, family, friends, pets, or practitioners who work with your body, I wish this for you often.

The Pain Body

No matter the type, pain is the feeling of distress. Physical pain is very tricky, as it is difficult to navigate. Being in constant pain can turn you into someone you don't even recognize. My pain came in the form of fear and not trusting in my body or its health. Physically I was afraid of losing my breath, dropping dead, or fainting (more so in public). I feared for my life and every breath for a very long period of time. However, experiencing constant or chronic physical pain is something entirely different. According to research from Harvard and published through the *Journal of Research and Pain Management*, doctors take women's complaints about chronic pain less seriously than the complaints of men. While it's unfortunate that medical discrimination is happening within the system, it means you must be very insistent when speaking to medical staff regarding pain. Make it clear that you need to be taken seriously. If you aren't, find someone else who will listen, test, and give the support you need.[12]

---

12. Anke Samulowitz, Ida Gremyr, Gunnel Hensign, "'Brave Men' and 'Emotional Women': A Theory-Guided Literature Review on Gender Bias in Health Care and Gendered Norms toward Patients with Chronic Pain." https://www.ncbi.nlm.nih.gov/pmc/articles/PMC5845507/.

How you approach your pain matters. We expand our pain bodies when we experience heartbreak, loss, and grief, as well as physical ailments that plague our body's natural operating system. When I think of a pain body, I think of a heaviness that brings everything else down. This can happen easily when we experience grief or get sick and our nervous system gets out of whack. What might start as a small area of pain can quickly spread like wildfire, and then everything goes down in flames. We can feel achy, heavy, lethargic, nervy/tingly, and uncomfortable to the touch. We begin to carry around what seems like a second body in our exact shape and size but it's heavier and less flexible and doesn't particularly enjoy movement.

Pain pathways are different from the pain body; they are more finite and definitive. There is actual research on the pain pathways in the body that report something like a highway of pain and nerve ache that travels in specific treads along the body. Once the pain pathways have been invoked from injury or cell damage, we have real issues that need to be addressed. The pain can persist even after whatever stimulus that caused the pain has been removed because the body figures how to create pain patterns and pathways that remain within our bodies even after the pain has been lessened or removed. One pathway works with our central nervous system (CNS, the brain and spinal cord) and is called "central sensitization," which can occur from a buildup of sensitivity to an area that may have been injury related. Pain of this type tends to leave an imprint in place even after whatever caused the problem has been removed, something like a pain echo. The pain that remains is the memory of the old pain, even though it is quite possible that it doesn't actually have a real correspondence with the nerve cells. In this situation, a person can still very much feel the pain as if it's still present, even if the person was told or shown that the pain was not real and should thus not be experienced any longer. This pain pathway can continue to create itself in its own image of pain. Isn't it wild that our bodies can be so crafty that they can continue to create pain in the old pain's image? Though this may sound scary, it leads us to the hope that if the body can create pain that isn't there, there is at least a possibility to get rid of it.

The other pain pathway we can experience is called "peripheral sensitization," which occurs after an injury, trauma, or damage to an area. In these situations, a person can now become highly sensitive to touch and heat. Where previously there would have not been pain in a specific area, the same amount of touch to the affected area can now cause significant pain. Imagine getting a burn on your arm and someone accidentally brushes up against that area. What used to be something harmless and simple now can become quite painful—even after recovery has occurred.

In the first response, the pain continues to be felt as pain without anything touching it. In the second, pain occurs when something touches the area even though it shouldn't technically lead to a pain response. Injuries can jolt the nervous system into reacting by unleashing chronic pain from the time of impact onward. Science is still unclear as to why some people experience acute pain after an injury that goes away, but others experience it as turning into chronic pain that seems to linger. For this secondary situation, the all too common approach to deal with the pain is through morphine or other opioid medications. Neuroscience research says that chronic pain is something like a "maladaptive memory." According to Dr. Yves De Koninck, professor of neuroscience at Université Laval in Quebec, Canada, chronic pain is the result of something that was embedded into the brain and nervous system upon infliction.[13] He has made the correlation between chronic pain and body memory, information that long-term body workers have also reported. Body memory, cellular memory, and muscle memory can lead to chronic pain. Medication is one way to deal with the pain because it allows us to be functional through it, but there are other healing practices that can help too. That said, these healing practices require a person to work with their bodies and go deep into the areas of the body/mind where the memory of the pain began so that it can be worked out. I realize this is easier said than done; rarely is healing this simple. But if reading that statement triggered you in any way, ask yourself: "Have I done any work around my emotional body to release my pain's deep-seated inflictions?" We must be willing to start right here exactly—this spot is our ground zero if we want to make any changes to the body and its association to a specific pain.

A group of researchers at New York University found that long-term memories connect to brain receptors and are felt through the central nervous system. However, when working with these old memories in a way to reduce or remove the pain patterns associated with them, there is a very brief moment between retrieving the memory from the body storage and feeling it. This finding offers an extremely small window of opportunity to interrupt the memory from being pulled and thus felt. The researchers found that if the feeling part of the memory can be removed, the body can then change as a result. The

---

13. Eleanor Nelson, "Teaching the Nervous System to Forget Chronic Pain," PBS+GPB NOVA NEXT (August 13, 2014). https://www.pbs.org/wgbh/nova/article/chronic-pain/.

pain and feeling pathway can be broken down and repaved. What they found was that a chemical called anisomycin can block the receptors activated by the neurons in order to keep the memory. Working on lab rats, they injected the chemical into the brains immediately following a trigger of a certain memory. When they did this, what they found was incredible … and a little frightening: Not only did they interrupt the rats' process of retrieving the memory, but apparently the memory was erased completely.[14]

I offer this study to show that even with chronic pain conditions, new findings are constantly being published that show that reversing and healing all sorts of conditions is possible—even some conditions that were once considered incurable. Remember as well that science is generally slower to catch up and verify the body's emotional and feeling components when it comes to any type of pain patterns. Certain hands-on healing or alternative healing practices might currently hold the keys that you are looking for. Be open to the avenues that have been shown to be successful in healing the conditions you need, no matter their form, so long as they are safe. Isn't it wonderful news that the pain body doesn't have to remain a pain body forever? Keep hope alive and continue your search.

How you approach your body and your healing is your responsibility. Physical and chronic pain can be debilitating and life wrecking, no doubt. I am in no way trying to minimize the anguish that accompanies the pain you might be experiencing. When you are angry, upset, and disappointed in whatever your body might be doing right now, it's okay to feel that way. Honor each feeling that comes up. When you're mad, be mad! Not everything is butterflies and rainbows all the time. Although I highly encourage positive dialogue within your body, I also know that if it's not coming from a real place, it really doesn't make the changes you need. So, feel it all—but don't get lost in it. Don't decide to live there and let those hard feelings start calling the shots. In the end, your mind is so much more influential than you might realize. We will go deeper into this during the emotional body section. What we can do with our mind can bring forth a whole wealth of new knowledge and healing.

---

14. Nathan Fried, "Lost in Translation: Without New Proteins, Chronic Pain Cannot Take Off. A first-in-class RNA decoy blocks PABP from attaching to messenger RNA, preventing translation and pain sensitization," Pain Research Forum. https://www.painresearchforum.org/news/92810-lost-translation-without-new -proteins-chronic-pain-cannot-take.

⌘ Practice: Between Retrieval of a Memory and Feeling the Pain

This little exercise comes from my dear friend, Stephen Watson. He wanted to simply take me out of whatever space I was in and help my mind realign into the present moment. When I did this simple practice, all I could think about was the study I mentioned earlier with the mice where the doctors created interference with the chronic pain pathways. To recap, there is a brief moment where the thoughts that retrieve a memory and the feeling associated with the pain of that memory can be disrupted. Give it a try and see if it works for you to help you notice that small window where the brain freezes up and has to rearrange its flow of thought. My personal feeling is that what you're doing in this exercise is making the same space that, if we were mice in the study, we'd receive the anisomycin injection.

Look around the room you are currently in. Make a mental note of every single item in the room that is yellow. Once you have done so, close your eyes and take a moment. Keeping your eyes closed, now try to think of anything in that room that was purple. See what that did? It tricked your mind and gave it a hiccup within your thought patterns for a single moment of time.

We can practice some of these things ourselves without having injections and still be able to mentally change up our patterns of thought that relate to pain. Begin to identify with that quick moment and see how you can better direct your thoughts with intention to help decrease the level of pain that is retrieved. The mind is powerful. Take that mental power and work with your inner hardwiring to lessen your internal experiences within your expressions of pain.

Learning how to turn a bad influence into something supportive and loving is a very tough road to find, and sticking to that road is even harder. But it is the road that leads to amazing new opportunities. What if you could get yourself to a place where your body can remember what it feels like to feel free? What if you can get to a place where you feel strong enough, confident enough, and comfortable enough to remind the inner workings of the cells, tissues, muscles, and memory to lock itself into complete health and freedom from pain? It *is* possible, and it begins right in this very moment when you agree to make it so.

Believing in your body, in your whole self, is where this starts. I'm not asking you to pretend your pain does not exist, because denial will tear this whole thing down. Your practice starts with the awareness and acceptance of the pain exactly as it is. When you do so, you're allowing that pain to be transmuted into something you can manage. You can do this. Your body does not rule your mind; in fact, it's the other way around. Give those cells and muscles a new conversation. There are options in all of our healing. Trust that this process will lead you to other avenues to heal your whole body.

⌘ Practice: Journaling with Your Pain

Time to take out your trusty journal. If you don't have one, now is as good a time as any to find one. I'm about to say something when it comes to pain and the practicing of living with pain—chronic, acute, or otherwise—that might at first make you audibly huff in disappointment for my simplicity and Pollyana attitude. I get it, but it needs to be said—and I'm going to defer to someone who lives with chronic pain, Sarah Anne Shockley, author of *The Pain Companion,* and that is this: "Make friends with your pain." Sarah was a guest on my radio show and we delved deep into this discussion. She taught me a great deal about the power of changing our relationship to our personal experiences of pain. It doesn't mean it goes away; it simply allows a shift to occur where you are more able to get it to a place that you can manage it more readily.

When the enemy no longer fulfills the "enemy" role, you can reassess and change it to become something more. In this case, pain can be reshaped into an annoying tag-along rather than an all-out enemy. As Sun Tzu says in the *Art of War,* "The supreme art of war is to subdue the enemy without fighting."[15] Change the game and the name of your pain. If it's acute and you've recently been hurt, involved in an accident, or the pain is not physical but emotional such as being betrayed or hurt feelings, then making friends out of the situation seems unlikely. In this case, don't make friends but make it a bygone instead. Give it a new name and make it become something you can either work with or acknowledge and release. Write its

---

15. Eric Jackson, "Sun Tzu's 31 Best Pieces of Leadership Advice," *Forbes,* May 23, 2014. https://www.forbes.com/sites/ericjackson/2014/05/23/sun-tzus-33-best-pieces-of-leadership-advice/#4e1223c95e5e.

name on paper. Burn it to release it from your hands or bury it in the ground if you intend it to blossom into something else. When it comes to conditions that involve chronic pain, making friends with your pain can actually change the level of pain you experience. Fighting against it gives it so much more power than figuring out a way to work with it. Write a letter to your pain and acknowledge it for exactly what it is and how it feels. But just like the secret shared in the breathing section of exhaling fully before allowing a new breath in, the same idea here applies: first write to your pain about all of your anger, frustration, and disappointment in its decision to move in with you. Don't hold anything back. Make space so that something new can enter into that place you just emptied.

Next, offer an olive branch to your pain. It is *your* pain, after all; it has decided to come and live with you. How will you choose to let it live? In a guest house that you visit from time to time? Will you have an arrangement where you acknowledge its presence enough so that it doesn't have to come knocking on your front door? Will it be down the street in a retirement community where you can visit on your own terms? Or do you want to keep it inside your home where you can keep your eye on it? It's up to you, but the most important thing to keep in mind is that you cannot afford to simply ignore the pain. Ignoring or denying the pain only gives it power. See it for what it is and feel it for what it is. Then give it the opportunity to shape-shift into something a little bit more useful for you. Write your way through this one.

✼ Practice: Working with Stones to Alleviate Pain

This exercise can work with physical pain, emotional pain, an excess of energy in the body, or whenever you need help to balance yourself. It is done while lying down. If you have a heavier stone such as a large obsidian (any of the obsidian family does best here: rainbow, green sheen, simple black, or snowflake), place this stone on the center of the chest, or over a physical area that has pain. Next, place a rose quartz stone above the obsidian on the center of the chest. The third stone is a clear quartz to be placed on the third eye or at the top of the head. First, begin with the dark stone that is over any pain area or lying on the chest below the rose quartz. Only focus on this stone. Place any unwanted pain, emotion, or energy into this stone—it's okay, the obsidian can take it. Breathe deeply as you send all of your unwanted expression into this stone. Give it all to the stone. Do this for as long as you need to until you feel a shift occur where you are not carrying quite so much inside anymore. Once you feel softer and lighter, begin to focus on the rose quartz at the heart center. Rose quartz is for unconditional love. Allow this energy to clean and clear your heart space. Finally, the clear quartz helps to protect, and clear the mind and body. Simply allow it to do its job. Surrender yourself completely when engaging in this practice. You could find rocks outside and do the same practice if you do not have these stones, but be sure that the stone that takes the unwanted energy is always the same stone. Do not mix them up and play around. Stones are sacred and incredibly powerful healing partners if you allow them to be. I engage in this personal practice so often that I truly don't know what I would do if I didn't have this to turn to in times of pain or strife.

The Pleasure Body

What comes up must come down. Where there is pain, there is pleasure nearby! It's just that sometimes pleasure likes to wear camouflage. Too many times when we get into discussions on healing, we tend to focus on the traumas that need to be healed. This is accurate but not complete. Everything we treat always has its counterpart. The pleasure body lives on the other side of the pain body. You don't have to totally overcome pain in order to experience pleasure. You can visit them both however equally you want to. I personally like a balance. Remember you are experiencing life through your one physical body.

Imagine if every part of your body felt energetically charged, comfortable, sensual, sacred, and balanced. Just as there are pain pathways that can travel throughout our bodies, so too are there pleasure pathways and secret spots from which we can pull to create something truly sublime. Pleasure lives inside us all, otherwise there would be no such thing as an orgasm! Understand that as I offer this section, although it does have a central focus on sexual energy and touch through your sacred sex areas, this is not at all the *only* way to experience pleasure.

One avenue to commune with your pleasure body is through thoughts, sounds, smells, taste, and by music. Notice we have five basic physical senses, but in order to use them to reach our pleasure body each must transform into something much higher than the basic energy that makes up the original principle. We were all born with the inherent right to be our own source of pain or pleasure. It really comes down to looking at the simple things with a new awareness of just how powerful their offerings really can be, and then allowing yourself to retreat into a space of pleasure. The way that we move our bodies can create so much satisfaction if given the right tools. Sacred dance, or any movements with intention to elevate the spirit is completely different than just getting out and exercising. There are certain things in life that are best experienced and enjoyed through the physical plane. You should not ever feel guilty allowing yourself to enjoy your life and the gifts that Spirit gave you.

Some people can get in touch with their pleasure bodies by using their body and breath to attain a multitude of healthy comforts from within. Whether working alone or with a partner, the breath is one of the most sacred instruments we have that allows us to experience supreme bliss. I once went to Toni Bergin's JourneyDance class, and I felt like my whole body exploded into a high that no drug could ever match—after my first class! I felt punch-drunk as love filled my entire being from the movements and the release of emotions. People were crying and hugging and rejoicing. This is a perfect example of the pleasure body and how we can achieve a level of bliss through physical movement combined with a spiritual pleasure.

Personal touch and pleasure are rarely discussed, but they are important. It's a very sacred practice (or it can be) to discover what your body is capable of. We become empowered from within in a multitude of ways when we learn how the body enjoys touch and pleasure. If you know how to reach climax on your own, you become more protective of your body and more deliberate in choosing who is allowed to come visit. Your body is your temple. It is the house of your soul. It's something we must protect, and nourish. If you are working with a partner, then touch and synchronized breath can be extremely powerful tools to experience pleasure and union as well.

Anything that makes your soul sing a little bit more is your ability to tap into your pleasure body. It's turning things that stimulate your senses into a more 4-D experience. Fundamentally, it's allowing yourself to enjoy whatever you are doing in a way that focuses on how good something feels. The hard part is really allowing ourselves to simply enjoy the good stuff. So many of us have deep-rooted conditioning that if we enjoy something, or hit a high part of our life, then surely the other shoe must drop. We have a hard time being present to the bliss that occurs for us in our lives. It's scary to let go and trust the Universe that the goodness we receive does not need to pair with tragedy. To change that conditioning requires the retraining of our old patterns and guilt systems to be more gluttonous, not with food per se, but with anything that feels really good. Don't be afraid to spend a little bit more time in pursuit of pleasures. If it wasn't meant to be enjoyed, it wouldn't be an option to have.

Connecting Through Energy and Intention

Obviously we can't discuss the pleasure body without the mention of the nervy and sensitive genital areas. Two very different forms of pleasure (breath and genitals) are experienced in one body from different ends. We can experience sublime highs through climax much the same way we can experience bliss through our breath and our intention. Sex is one thing, but sacred sex takes the experience of mingling energies to an entirely different level. This sacred area doesn't have to just be about sex nor does it in any way need to include another person.

⌘ Practice: Solitary Sex

Learning how your body responds to pleasure is vitally important and requires a personal practice. It's the intention behind the practice that is the most valuable part of this exploration. Practicing self-pleasure with the intention of turning sexual energy into manifesting power is something everyone can be privy to. Pairing thoughts and intention with any part of pleasure play can be very powerful. To explore without guilt and learn about the magic and wisdom that your body holds is an important first step in gathering your personal power and learning how to harness your energy. It also creates a boundary within oneself and the body. Once you know the power and wisdom of your body and how it responds to stimulation and pleasure, you may be less likely to give it away for less than what you could bring to the table by yourself. It becomes a practice in learning how to worship in our own temple, and naturally we begin to protect it fiercely. There is incredible power to manifest through your intention and energy that can turn into powerful realities once you get a handle on how to work with them through this space.

✿ PRACTICE: SINGULAR PRACTICE TO CONNECT ENERGY THROUGH INTENTION

If you need to come into a silent, calm space using your breath and your intention, a great place to begin is by placing one hand over your heart and the other below the ribs and above the navel at the solar plexus. Close your eyes and imagine a multicolored healing rainbow coming from the palm of one hand into the palm of the other. Allow the rainbow of colors to connect from the backside of each hand to formulate an entire circle of multicolored energy circulating between your heart (space of love) and your solar plexus (place of knowing). Breathe deeply into the colors and connect the energy and colors circulating with your breathing pattern. Inhale slowly through the nose for a count of four, exhale through the mouth for a count of six or eight. Continue this practice for as long as it takes to remove you from whatever is in the outside world.

✿ PRACTICE: PARTNER PRACTICE TO CONNECT ENERGY THROUGH INTENTION

Sit facing your partner with crossed legs, or with the smaller partner sitting over the seated lap with their legs wrapped around the larger partner's. Begin by placing each right hand on the other person's heart space in the center of the chest. Next place each left hand on top of your partner's hand that is over your own heart space. It creates a figure-8 infinity symbol between the outgoing and ingoing hands. Close your eyes and bring the foreheads together to touch. Together, exhale through the nose. Breathe through the nose for both the inhale and exhale together so as not to overpower with breathing out of the mouth onto the other person. The breathing should be slow but complete, fluid, and silent. Inhale either for two or four counts and exhale for four, six, or eight counts. Try to use those counting numbers as a suggestion and don't count the breathing when working with a partner. Instead, try to be the one to set the pace of the breath, or follow your partner's pattern if that's the only way to get the breaths to match up. Inhale at the same time, and exhale at the same time. Bring your foreheads together and close your eyes. Keep the hands at the heart space. Stay in this space for as long as it takes to connect the energies together. Let it create a new experience and go with it, or gently release and separate when you are ready. It's entirely the choice between those engaged in this practice. Take it all in and be completely present to yourself and your partner in thoughts, breaths, and bodies. Take great delight in experiencing this level of pleasure. Ride that wave wherever it goes. If you feel compelled to speak, do so. If you are guided to take this into a more physical experience with your partner, keep the breathing and intention. This is a powerful way to connect deeply into another person and bring the energies of the two into one strong space. It is also a wonderful way to manifest your desires and intentions into the physical world. State your intention before starting this practice so that the energy can morph into something greater. Stating an intention with a singular or partner practice can transmute the desired intentions into reality. It moves the energy through the bodies and into the ethers. It is a powerful addition to the practices.

Whether connecting with a partner or connecting simply with ourself, it's important that we take time to explore the pleasure body both intimately and simply. Taking notice of the simple pleasures in life is paramount in changing our paradigm to one of cultivating a life of gratitude and love. That starts from inside ourselves and then transforms our exterior world around us. Do not delay pleasure of any kind any longer—you deserve to enjoy your life and you are not getting this day back again, so be all in and let yourself enjoy the ride.

Part III
The Emotional Body

Our bodies respond to the way we think, feel, behave, and express. Feel all of it. The messy, the beautiful, the anguish, the excitement, the losses, and the loves. Feel it all and hold back nothing. Taking charge of your emotional health can free your body and your mind in ways that might only look like a dream for now. Make friends with your emotions and use them for good. I believe in you. Keep going!

Chapter 6

Mental and Emotional Therapies

The body's emotional layer requires a totally different treatment protocol for addressing imbalance than the physical layer does. This chapter covers your emotional and mental state of well-being. The emotional body is a layer that guides us to the healthy pathways in the body, mind, and soul, to include thoughts, feelings, and behaviors toward the self and others. How you feel about situations, how you handle the life you've created, and how you respond to outside influences all play a role in the way the emotional body is affected. It's the voice inside your head that when in balance repeats healthy and positive affirmative dialogue but when out of balance can create a state of total chaos. We will explore in this chapter the various practitioners and therapies who can help with your mental state, as it's important to know the differences between each practice. Our emotional state sets the stage for our overall health; without a healthy mind the body cannot achieve any level of optimal health. Luckily, there are many places and people you can see to help you get a strong handle on your emotional health and ability to cope with life's stressors.

On the topic of emotional health, the American Psychological Association states:

… Emotional health can lead to success in work, relationships, and health. In the past, researchers believed that success made people happy. Newer research reveals that it's the other way around. Happy people are more likely to work toward goals, find the resources they need, and attract others with their energy and optimism—key building blocks of success.[16]

Psychology

Psychology is the discipline of science that studies and observes the mind as it functions and behaves. A psychologist works with your behavior patterns when you are out of balance but does not prescribe medication. Their expertise is in understanding the mind's cognitive skills and function. There are many different psychologists out there; each usually has a specific practice of therapy in which they specialize. Finding the right match for what you are in need of will be a huge factor in determining the right therapist for you.

Psychotherapy

A psychotherapist helps a client with behaviors and helps them overcome the associated problems in their life due to those behaviors. The aim of this practice is to help improve a person's general well-being and mental health. Psychotherapists work with behaviors, addictions, and compulsions. There are more than a thousand different practice techniques under the umbrella of psychotherapy. Some psychotherapists work with families or groups while others stick to individual client practices.

Clinical Psychology

A clinical psychologist is a much more specialized practitioner. The focus is usually on assessment, diagnoses, and treatments of mental illness or disabilities. Any practice with the "-ology" suffix indicates that the practice is mind-based therapy; medication is not prescribed under any psychological practice, even in clinically based ones. The most commonly treated disorders in this practice include anxiety, depression, schizophrenia, and post-traumatic stress disorders. Even if you see a clinical psychologist, the focus is still on a patient's mental behaviors; they will usually offer ways to cope with more difficult situations. Often, they commonly work in conjunction with psychiatrists.

---

16. American Psychological Association, "Emotional Health," https://www.apa.org/topics/emotion.

Neuropsychology

In the practices of neuroscience and neuropsychology, doctors are more apt to study the cognitive, emotional, and behavioral effects more associated with brain-based conditions. This is a more evidence-based and clinical practice; many times, neuropsychologists will specifically work with individuals who have a malfunction in the brain such as autism, stroke, dementia, or brain injury or damage.

Psychiatry

A psychiatrist is a medical doctor who assesses, diagnosis, and treats mental illness through the prescription of medication. If you hear the word "psychiatrist," know that you are going to someone specifically for the purpose of getting a prescription to help you in your functioning. The important distinction to make here is that the mind and the brain are not the same thing. The brain is an organ, so sometimes it is necessary to treat the brain chemistry by correcting its off-balance chemical makeup via medical intervention. A good psychiatrist will also prescribe a particular therapy with a psychologist in conjunction with medication so that you can learn better coping skills and behavior patterns more than just balancing the chemicals in the brain. If you need medication, remember that there is no shame in this game. Do not let people make you feel guilty or bad for getting the help you need. It is no one's right to make decisions for you when it comes to your health and healing.

Child Psychology

If you are looking to find someone to help your child, you may need to see a child specific practice both in psychology and psychiatry. A child's brain development is extremely different in the first ten years of life than at any other age. The warp speed of synapses that grow and build are something really amazing within that time frame. This is why getting early intervention is the key in helping children overcome obstacles within their behaviors and brain development. A child psychologist and a child psychologist who can administer tests and diagnose a child are not exactly the same thing. When looking for getting a diagnosis, it is a specific child psychologist who only tests for the purpose of diagnosing is your best bet. Then seeing someone who specializes in working with children according to the specific diagnosis is a most successful formula to follow. A diagnostic child psychologist and a child psychologist who is in practice for therapies are two different practitioners. It is important to differentiate the two. Some people see developmental pediatricians for the diagnosis and then find the psychologist for the execution of behavior modification according to the findings.

Child Neuropsychologist

If you are working with a child specific neuropsychologist their testing will vary widely from an educational psychologist for diagnosis and testing. A Neuropsychologist with children will assess cognition, behavior, memory and attention, learning and processing, speed of learning and processing as well as abstract behaviors. They study information that is more linked to the brain structures to help provide information that might impact areas of difficulty for the child in all aspects of life.

Educational Psychologist

If you are working with a child, seeing an educational psychologist is specifically necessary for the education system only. They are concerned with how a child behaves, learns, and processes information with regard strictly to school work. Their testing is totally different than a test through a Neuropsychologist for the same child. It will provide very different answers for that child. Their tests will center around academic function, history, academic skills, intellect, and conduct. (This is the same with a Pediatric Occupational Therapist for the school verses private practice. You would see them for different assessments).

Talk Therapy/Cognitive Therapies

This book's appendix offers a chart that summarizes what this chapter covers. In this section, the emotional chart features the various doctors and therapists as well as actual therapies that work in conjunction with them. When looking for any therapy, refer to the top of the chart for the kind of practitioner you should look for and be sure that they are specialized in the method of therapy you have interest in pursuing.

Emotional Imbalances

The body's emotional aspect is related to thoughts as well as behavior patterns. The way we experience our lives, process our environments, and behave in the world are all related to this aspect. This section covers mood and mental illness as well as personal relationships.

Mental-Emotional Imbalances

The mental part is our mind and the emotional part is our feelings.[17] For many of us, how we think and how we feel may be difficult to manage. There are actually two hundred classified types of mental illness recognized in the medical community that affect our emotional health. Some, such as general anxiety and depression, are more commonly classified as mood disorders than mental illnesses. They are different in terms of labeling, diagnostics, and treatments. Personally, I don't like the term *mental illness*; I prefer *emotional imbalance*. I'll list the primary emotional imbalance categories as well as a brief offering of examples within each particular category. The primary categories include:

Anxiety disorders: generalized anxiety disorder (GAD), social anxiety, obsessive-compulsive (OCD), post-traumatic stress disorder (PTSD), and social phobias

Mood disorders: depression, bipolar disorder, borderline personality disorder

Schizophrenia and other psychotic disorders: schizoid personality disorder

Dementia: Alzheimer's disease, trauma to the head/brain, Parkinson's, HIV, substance-induced dementia

Eating disorders: anorexia, bulimia nervosa, and binge-eating disorders[18]

These often require medical treatment with a team of both a psychiatrist and psychologist. This is the combination of medication and cognitive therapies. It is important to note the different options and therapies for healing. There are so many out there, the key is to find the right combination for your healing.

Cognitive therapy comes in two parts: (1) finding the right avenue of treatment, and (2) finding the right therapist to take you through it. Finding the best therapist is the

---

17. Silvana Galderisi, Andreas Heinz, Marianne Kastrup, Norman Sartorius, "Toward a new definition of mental health," *World Psychiatry* June 4, 2015. DOI: 10.1002/wps.20231.

18. Mental Health, "5 Types of Mental Illness and Disability," UPMC HealthBeat, May 27, 2015. https://share.upmc.com/2015/05/5-types-of-mental-illness-and-disability/.

more important of the two in my opinion. If you don't have a strong rapport and a healthy respect for how they work with you, keep looking. This is about your healing, and if it isn't a match, don't try to force it to be. As mentioned before, the various therapists in this field tend to practice with one specialty for behavior modification. Some of these include:

Hypnotherapy

There are many applications of hypnotherapy. It is used as an adjunct along with other forms of psychological and medical treatments. Hypnotherapy can be used to help a person recover from phobias, anxiety, sleep issues, smoking cessation, weight loss, bad habits or undesirable behaviors, sexual dysfunction, learning disorders, relationship issues, pain management, digestive disorders, skin issues, gastrointestinal side effects, chemotherapy, pregnancy, and more.

Hypnotherapy does not put you all the way under so that you are not aware of what happens in your session. It helps to guide you into a very relaxed state of consciousness so that the new programming can plant roots deep and grow with you. It's common for sessions to be recorded and to receive a copy of the recording to listen to again and again to help retrain your mind. You are aware of everything around you but are less attached to your body and thoughts during the session. The hypnotherapist will work with you prior to the session itself to help with what you are wanting to see happen with this treatment. It is a very comfortable, calm, and soft approach to healing that yields big results.

Regression Therapy

This is a form of hypnosis where a person can go back in time to when they were younger or even a baby in order to visit the place where the trauma originally occurred. There is also past life regression therapy that can take you back to the lives you have led before this life in order to help clear karma and understand behaviors that present themselves in your current life that you can't trace through this particular incarnation as the source. Dr. Brian Weiss is often considered the father of past-life regression work, and his book *Many Lives, Many Masters* is a treasure that many still use to this day.

Eye Movement Desensitization Reprocessing (EMDR)

EDMR is a form of psychotherapy that has extensive research behind it that seeks to treat the sources of trauma such as PTSD, anxiety, phobias, grief, panic attacks, pain disorders, body dysmorphic disorders, personality disorders, sexual or physical abuse, dissociative disorders, and more. This protocol pulls from many different methods of treatment approaches and is considered very effective.

EMDR directly affects the way in which the brain process information. When a person experiences trauma, the sounds, images, smells, and feelings associated with the trauma are essentially frozen in time, which can have a long-lasting effect on a person and the way in which they relate to the world around them. It affects personal relationships with everyone in the person's life going forward. EMDR has a similar reaction to what occurs when a person enters REM sleep. It has been proven to improve the way a person sees and experiences the trauma once they've cleared the neuroactivity around the original traumatic event.

Cognitive Behavioral Therapy (CBT)

CBT aims to help with unhealthy behaviors and improve a person's ability to regulate their emotions. This is an area where developing coping skills is a primary goal. CBT is considered to be a short-term therapy (usually around twenty sessions), as it is a problem-specific approach to wellness and behavior modifications. The idea behind it is that the way that someone thinks and interprets life experiences affects how they behave in response. Once a person learns how to better accept life situations that arise, they can put those coping skills to use and handle situations in a healthier, more positive way.

Dialectical Behavioral Therapy (DBT)

DBT is an evidence-based form of treatment originally intended to work specifically with individuals who have borderline personality disorder. Later research has shown that it also helps to work around additional mood disorders such as self-harming behaviors, substance abuse, suicidal ideation, bipolar disorder, PTSD, bulimia, and binge eating. The treatment approach focuses on four key areas: (1) mindfulness (2) distress tolerance (3) emotion regulation and (4) interpersonal effectiveness.

DBT is designed to be used in both one-on-one therapy, as well as DBT skills groups where patients work together as a group to share their experience and offer support to other group members. As a group, homework is assigned. The group sessions generally last for two hours at a time for a length of six months, meeting once a week. Those with borderline personality disorder experience extreme negativity with their emotions and all their relationships—friends, partners, family. The therapist in this case will work with the negative behaviors and teach the person coping skills and new thinking patterns that can be put in place to change the way they view themselves and others. For this reason, group work is helpful as it allows people to support each other as they try to change their very strongly imprinted sets of behaviors. DBT supports an outlook of "both/and" attitudes instead of "either/or" (the latter of which people with borderline personality disorder commonly have).[19]

Acceptance and Commitment Therapy (ACT)

This form of psychotherapy stems from traditional cognitive therapy practice. In it, people learn to accept their feelings in response to life's situations instead of avoiding and denying their emotions. Accepting that certain feelings and emotions associated with life experiences should not prevent them from living their best life moving forward. This is a straightforward approach that requires personal action. A person will work with their inner dialogue and change the self-talk behaviors to a more objective and positive dialogue. This helps to work with conditions such as chronic pain, diabetes, substance abuse, depression, bipolar disorder, psychosis, test and social anxieties, obsessive-compulsive disorder, and general stress.

Talk Therapy

Talk therapy allows a patient to talk freely about what they have been feeling in their lives. This is a form of cognitive therapy that is more free-form. Sometimes people need someone to talk to who is not necessarily a partner, family member, or friend who can offer healthy and helpful responses or simply just listen without making judgment. Also called insight therapy, the idea is that by talking through certain things, the person may

---

19. "Dialectical Behavioral Therapy," *Psychology Today*. https://www.psychologytoday.com/us/therapy-types /dialectical-behavior-therapy.

gain insight into their behavioral patterns. In this practice, patients learn about themselves through sharing whatever is going on in their lives. It sounds simple, but talk is a wonderful form of therapy. I personally sought talk therapy when a certain situation in my life had become all-consuming and I didn't want to burden my friends or family talking about the same thing over and over again. It provides a safe space to put it all out there and hopefully gain insight into better ways to detach from whatever issues are becoming overwhelming. Other therapies include talk and behavior modifications for an individual, group, or as family therapy.

Biofeedback

Biofeedback as a clinical practice is a technique that a person can learn to control the body's responses such as heart rate, skin temperature, and blood pressure. These things are generally controlled by the nervous system and are considered to be controlled involuntarily, not through a specific practice or effort. Biofeedback is a systematic approach to help someone gain control over responses to their environment such as getting excited, nervous, or in response to exercise. The biofeedback technique aims to teach the participant how to gain control by harnessing the power of the mind to control the body.

In a biofeedback session, electrodes are placed on the skin and sensors for the fingers can also be used. These sensors and electrodes monitor a person's heart rate, breathing rate, body temperature, blood pressure, and muscle movements. Because stress affects each of these functions in a big way, this practice is used to help a person learn to calm themselves down from a deep inner level in order to affect each of these body responses as they occur in real time. A biofeedback therapist will help a person to learn to work with their stress responses and practice deeper relaxation techniques as they learn to control their body. People seek out biofeedback to help with issues such as migraines, incontinence, high blood pressure, and chronic pain.

Practices for Psychosomatic (Mind/Body) Healing
Quantum Physics Biofeedback

This is a tough one to explain, because it sounds really out there. I have received this particular healing twice in my life from different practitioners. During the process, a sensor strap is hooked up to your ankles, wrists, and around your head. The device used for it is so sophisticated that it goes all the way to your DNA and can tell you anything that your body has come in contact with. It can tell you why you have the emotions that you do, what you are lacking nutritionally, what parts of your body are out of balance, and what you can do to restore them.

The cost of the equipment roughly equals the price of a new car, and I was surprised how accurate and detailed this machinery was with its results. I recommend that someone seek this biofeedback in situations where no one else can figure out what is wrong. No one should ever be without answers about their body or health. There is always something that can provide the answers. Look in the holistic community to find someone who works with this machine.

Sophrology

Until I interviewed the author of the book *The Life-Changing Power of Sophrology,* by Dominique Antiglio, I had never heard of this practice. Formally, this practice was created by neuropsychiatrist professor Alfonso Caycedo and is a method that allows people to connect the body and the mind via breathing and specialized mindset practices. Although widely practiced throughout Europe (Spain especially), it is not well known in the United States. Sophrology can be taught to any person to help with a multitude of emotional imbalances, and the treatment is very simple and effective. The name for the practice comes from: *sos,* "harmony," *phren,* "consciousness or spirit," *logos,* the science or study of—*sophrology* is thus "the science of consciousness in harmony."[20] Looking into sophrology, my own personal take on it is that it's like a single practice that combines my twenty years of studying various healing subjects simplifying them in such a way that becomes accessible to everyone. It's brilliant and a wonderful practice to incorporate if you are feeling stressed, anxious, depressed, or generally out of sync.

The Rosen Method

Founded by Marion Rosen, who has seventy years of experience as a physical therapist and body worker, this method is the combined result of her practice and knowledge. She created this psychosomatic practice to use movement and bodywork to help people achieve a new sense of health. Rosen works with specific muscles and body movements combined

---

20. Dominique Antiglio, *The Life-Changing Power of Sophrology* (New York: New World Library, 2018), 35.

with an emotional awareness to help create a dynamic treatment that helps the whole body to balance itself. In addition to creating the bodywork practice, she also created a specific movement class set to music where people can engage in relaxing movements in a group setting. A Rosen method practitioner has studied hundreds of hours through the institute in order to be able to treat according to this method of work.

The Feldenkrais Method

This powerful method uses the mind to help relax the body. Developed by Moshe Feldenkrais in the mid-twentieth century, this practice is considered a somatic education course to help the brain and body reorganize to higher levels of being. The practice encourages slow motions with mental clarity and intention to help increase flexibility, range of motion, perception of self, and sensitivity to the world within and around us all. It is a direct link to the perception of what the mind believes one can do, and then using guided imagery and intention to help one realize that the body is not nearly as limited as originally believed. The practice is soft and gentle yet powerful.

Chapter 7
Foundations of Emotions and Personal Relationships

I have found there to be nothing basic about the approach to primal human emotions. In this chapter we will discuss the differing opinions on how many central core emotions exist. There are several feeling and emotion charts out there for you to use, and they are a wonderful tool to better help you identify with your feelings. I strongly encourage you to do a little searching on your own to find the emotional pattern chart that you resonate with should you need one.

Ekman's Feeling Wheel

Psychologist Dr. Paul Ekman has stated that the most commonly held belief is that there are six basic emotions according to facial expressions: happiness, sadness, fear, anger, surprise, and disgust.[21]

Plutchik's Wheel of Emotion

Another famous doctor, Dr. Robert Plutchik (also an American psychologist), theorizes there are eight primary emotions: joy, sadness, trust, disgust, fear, anger, surprise, and anticipation. Plutchik created the wheel of emotion based on this theory. In it are eight

---

21. Neal Burton, "What Are Basic Emotions?" *Psychology Today,* June 21, 2019 https://www.psychologytoday .com/us/blog/hide-and-seek/201601/what-are-basic-emotions.

primary emotions followed by ten postulates (defined as the truth of something as a basis for reasoning).[22]

A Breakthrough?

Recent studies out of the University of Glasgow have offered a new challenge to the six-emotion model—there might just be four expressive patterns. Dr. Rachael Jack and her team developed software to generate a range of different face movement patterns by tracking the muscles of facial expression. They asked participants from different cultures and categorized each face movement by emotion. The four latent patterns they discovered came from an analysis of more than sixty different emotions such as cheerfulness, terror, unhappiness, and shame. They then analyzed the relationship between the face movement patterns (muscles of facial expression) and the participants' responses to mathematically model the specific face movement patterns. They looked at how the participants in different cultures associate with these different emotion categories. By analyzing the resulting set of more than sixty facial expression models, they discovered four latent expressive patterns that correspond to smiling, pouting, scowling, and wide-eyed gasping. Of the original six primary emotions of happiness, sadness, fear, anger, surprise, and disgust, anger and disgust as well as fear and surprise share the same characteristics and don't register until later on. According to Dr. Jack: "What our research shows is that not all facial muscles appear simultaneously during facial expressions, but rather develop over time supporting a hierarchical biologically-basic to socially-specific information over time."[23]

Feelings versus Emotions

There are many discrepancies between what we consider to be feelings and emotions. Through research, I've found that emotions are experienced physically and can be measured by things such as brain activity, blood flow, facial expressions, and even body positions. Feelings, on the other hand, are experienced through the mental process and therefore cannot be measured as specifically. In my opinion, it doesn't matter all that much whether we identify an experience as a feeling or an emotion; when it comes to the way

22. Burton, "Basic Emotions."

23. BBC News,"All human behavior can be reduced to 'four basic emotions'," BBC.com, February 3, 2014. https://www.bbc.com/news/uk-scotland-glasgow-west-26019586.

our body feels things, I prefer the term *experience* over the fine distinctions of thoughts, feelings, or emotions.

Emotions and Poison

As I see it, the emotional body does not give context only to the mind. I prefer to focus instead on the mind/body connection. Everything perceived through mental awareness and emotional depth is equally experienced through the entire body. The way you perceive your truths, process them, and express yourself through those truths are an integral part of the whole.

When it comes to our emotional health, I strongly believe that the emotions that are not processed and released tend to be the root cause of dis-ease. While genetics and life-style factors affect our health, we can easily discount how powerful the emotional piece is to the whole. Because my specialty is emotional release work through hands-on body work, I have a different perspective with regard to emotions and how they can affect the body. When left beneath the surface, they can create a host of illnesses within the body that likely will end up labeled under many diagnoses that still cover up the core truth. By acknowledging your emotional body, you can recover your power and reverse many illnesses that present as strictly physical. It's never one over the other, physical over emotional. You must not dismiss one of these aspects. One can be the primary root of the dis-ease, but both are powerful players in creating imbalance within the system. Both must be approached and treated equally to restore balance.

It is interesting (and rather disappointing) to note that very few body-related events can be nailed down as *X definitely causes Y*. What causes something may never be fully understood, so it follows that the cure will also never be a one-size-fits-all or a one-script protocol—it's always a combination of factors from different sources. Both the original causes and the liberation of illness have firm footing in our bodies' emotional layer. To discount this in any way is potentially damaging for your healing. Body healing through the use of emotional release is often done through hands-on energy work. Touching the physical body with a particular practice and intention allows us to release and remove the embedded emotions within the tissues.

When not being expressed, validated, and processed, emotions can turn on you. They bury down deep, releasing some sort of *stink gas* (that's a technical term!) as they burrow in. That stink gas becomes the toxic waste and poison that deposits itself into the tissues of your body. From there, a garden of rotten, putrid pain and anguish begins to grow. Yes, the gardens of the body can be glorious *or* poisonous. It's up to us to plant and grow wisely. We must grow them with wisdom and deliberation. Tending to our own gardens is something that needs to be taught (or re-taught) in a healthier context if we wish to reap the best fruits and flowers. If only more of us were taught in school how to handle our feelings, emotions, thoughts, and behaviors in a way that yields healthy outcomes. If you are offered these things, it likely came from really incredible parents or a great therapist. We need to be taught better skills in order to change the way we play life's game.

An Oncology Referral

I have been blessed to witness seeing someone who had a certain type and stage of cancer whose body was resisting the chemotherapy be able to accept the treatment once they released the excruciating emotional pain she had been avoiding. She was able to allow her body to heal herself through the release of the emotion embedded into the area beneath. This was done in conjunction with the physical treatments that were necessary to save her life. Her oncologist sent her to me to help her body accept the treatment she needed to save her life. Together, we uncovered the seed down deep under the area where the cancer was growing. As with many cancers that develop in the reproductive areas, there is a reason to look into history of sexual abuse. This is *not* to say in any form or fashion that if you or someone you know has issues in this area, I am pointing fingers and asking you to look for things that are not there; there are no hard and fast rules of any kind. What I am pointing out is that when it comes to a body disruption, especially in the more sensitive reproductive areas for men and women, it is valuable to explore first to rule out that particular emotional component.

When the woman was just a toddler, an older male member of her family chose to explore his curiosities through her body without her consent or understanding. She did not even remember this had happened to her until much later in life. Sadly, it wasn't until he made a big life change and expressed his regret and apology that the information was relayed to her. He came to her presenting this information and immediately asking for forgiveness. After receiving this news, it was a very short amount of time before she developed cancer in her ovaries. The damage was done—the cognitive power area (the mind) could manifest any action it needed in order to express the pain, trauma, shame, and guilt that accompanied his vile acts. This time, however, her body responded with a very serious, life-threatening disease.

It was through our emotional release session that I could help her to see the innocence of her child self. Whatever happened was not her fault. She began to cry so intensely with her whole body that I pulled a trash can up to the table in case she needed to vomit. Her letting out these emotions involved every cell, muscle, and tissue memory she had stowed away but was now coming out at once. I continued with my hands on her, bringing through her the mental imagery that allowed her to release the shame her body had locked into itself and held on to so tightly. The session was between two and three hours long; we could not stop until it was complete—a fully body release so exhausting that she could barely stand upon completion. It was an incredibly intense session and one that I will treasure for all of my life. I am honored to have been a part of it.

To our profound surprise and gratitude, the following week she went back to the oncologist. This time, however, her body no longer resisted the treatment as it had before. To date, she is now in year ten of remission. Her powerful healing came from the same exact place the illness grew from, within herself. From that same deep place inside herself, she allowed herself to heal and release the pain. In turn, her body released and reversed the illness that it had created. This is a dramatic, wild story of miracles and amazing healing, and it shows exactly how our emotions are related to physical treatment. Both were necessary to save this woman's life.

When she celebrates her birthday every year, the woman sends me a note saying that she will never forget the role I played in her story of life. But the truth is that it was never me—I was simply the conduit for Spirit to work through. Ultimately, it was the decision within her own body to allow itself to heal, and so she did. I also hope your takeaway from this story is that *you* also have incredible power to heal yourself and set yourself free to live your life to the fullest. Everything and anything are possible.

Personal Relationships

A great part of our emotional body comes down to the relationships we have with ourselves and others. How we connect with those around us whether as a child, parent, friend, or lover affects our emotional layer exponentially. Every person who caused you pain or built you up has a direct effect on your emotional body. When we lose a partner, a loved one, or a pet, it takes an enormous toll on our emotional body. When we find a partner, find a new friend, have a child, or get a pet, this too can enhance our emotional body in the most glorious ways. Remember too that relationships are not just partners but also the many different dynamics between ourselves and others. For our purposes here, I offer the best advice based on the work I do with people and their emotional bodies. I hope it will be helpful and supportive to you.

Parent/child

Not every person who needs to heal their emotional body experienced trauma as children. There are a great many people who had wonderful families and homes. Some people consider their mom, dad, brother, or sister to be their greatest support system and the place they always return to in order to feel restored in their soul. I personally had wonderful and loving parents and siblings. I loved my childhood and treasure it. My worst trauma was in the loss of the best father anyone could have. He was my greatest supporter and I miss him terribly every day. Even though my home was full of love, it was my dad who had my back the way I needed someone to have my back. Removing that support taught me a lot of hard-earned lessons on how to become my own best friend. I'll be honest and say that I became the typical girl with daddy issues. Who wouldn't?

Many of us grew up in homes that did not always confirm that we are strong, healthy, capable people who can do anything we set our minds to. Too many children were abused physically, verbally, and/or sexually. There are a great many people out in the world who need serious support in the way of psychological counseling and (if comfortable to receive) hands-on healing as well. If this at all pertains to you, let me say this: You are a worthy, lovable person who never deserved that sort of treatment. It was never your fault. You deserve healing and freedom from the bondage that you did not create. I am so sorry if any of this happened to you. No one ever has the right to put their hands on you without your permission. Please seek help to learn how to free yourself and change the path ahead. You deserve all the goodness and love that life has to offer. You are worthy and you are loved.

⌘ Practice: Parent/Child Relationship

When it comes to family, the best thing you can do is keep the lines of honesty and humility open. If you have been keeping secrets from your family, now is the time to share them and free yourself. Ask for help if you need help. If you have an amazing family or an amazing family member, then please be open and give them the gratitude they deserve. Don't ever assume a child just "knows" they are loved and appreciated. Share it. Say it often. Never miss the opportunity to share your love with the ones you trust the most.

Friendships

How many friends have we had throughout our lives that we thought would always be in our lives but are not anymore? Some friendships are meant to last a lifetime, while others come and go. We line up energetically and then tend to fall away when we or they make a shift that is no longer in alignment with the other. Who we match with is a reflection of where we are during each stage of our lives. Many friends come from sports teams, exercise classes, school, work, or who your children go to school with. There are friendships that help to lift us up and friendships that are ride or die. There are times when you find that a friendship you've had for a long time no longer feels good to you. Sometimes you make a shift that doesn't match the other person, so they leave your life... and sometimes it's you who leaves their life.

The most important thing that you can do if any of your relationships are shifting is to always be clear, kind, and honest. Don't make big decisions without consulting the other person. Try to give them a chance to express themselves. Make a mutual choice together based on the realities of where you are in your lives. Nothing is worse than having a close friend leave our lives without the respect to say why they are choosing to leave. It is cowardly, cruel, and is no reflection of the time you had with each other. The importance of mutual choice goes for both friendships and partner relationships. I've personally experienced both in which the person left without being able to be honest and own up to the part they played. I have no respect for that. As well, I've also withheld my feelings about something and simply stepped back from people after seeing behaviors that told me clearly that when it would come to the big stuff, I wouldn't be able to trust them fully. Being honest and up front about how you are feeling within any given situation is difficult, but you owe it to your relationships to be respectful of the time you've both put in before making any moves without letting them know why. My advice for friendships is do not expect from any friend more than you are willing to give. Be honest, be fair, and above all, be kind.

Friendships are some of our most glorious connections, and we need them in our lives. If you find yourself fighting often with friends, I suggest working with a therapist on behavior patterns and learning to take responsibility for your feelings and behaviors. Do not ever lie to your friends or loved ones. I know too many people who make up silly little lies to get out of things when if they just owned up, it would clean up a lot easier. I have an important personal rule that saves me a lot of grief, and it can save you too: If you lie to me, you will be removed from my life. I won't lie to you, and I won't allow you to lie to me three times. That said, I may not always offer up how I'm feeling freely. If asked, I will always tell my truth. I will not line up with people who aren't the same way.

⌘ Practice: The Stop and Share

I received a nugget of wisdom from my dear friend Ashli Callaway (spiritual counselor) in a conversation we had recently that was so powerful and simple that I thought everyone should hear it: She said to me that over the years we have collectively done a disservice to our relationships when we were not true to ourselves and weren't honest in the moment when something hurt us. She said that she works with her child on sharing her feelings in the moment they happen because she wants her child to feel empowered while sharing how she feels.

The next time someone says something hurtful to you (even if they didn't realize it was hurtful), be still; hold the space in the moment; and simply, kindly, and honestly say: "That really hurt my feelings" or "It embarrassed me when you said this to me in front of other people." It gathers the energy, honors it, disposes of it, and creates a wholly different dynamic within our relationships. If we immediately stop and share our feelings, it can prevent the days of festering and obsessing on how something affected us. The way my friend presented it was soft, kind, and I believe it holds the power to shut down any fighting tendencies. It would be very difficult to yell back at someone who simply, softly, and kindly said, "You hurt me." What more is there to say to that other than "I'm sorry"? Our strength is in our honesty. It will only create stronger foundations within our relationships.

Partner relationships

Who we choose as love partners is a direct reflection on what we feel we deserve. We are capable of experiencing the level of happiness and love to the same level that we can experience the depths of darkness and pain. That emotional energy can move just as deeply in both directions depending on what we allow in our bodies and in our lives, so choose wisely. Going through a breakup is something that can be devastating and last for a really long time. The truth is, I hope that at some point in your life you've had your heart broken. Why? Because I think when it comes to love relationships, those experiences are necessary in order for your soul to grow. To put it another way, those heartbreakers from the past were actually big openers into who you are becoming and what you are no longer willing to accept. They were (or are still) a chance for you to grow beyond what makes you feel anything less than loved and accepted exactly as you are. Lord knows I didn't always make good choices before I met my life partner, nor was I always a partner who exhibited behavior I could be proud of. Like most things in life, there was never a strictly one-sided fault unlike what we usually describe. I am grateful for most of the experiences, but I'd be lying if I said I was grateful for all of them! But more than any heartbreak, I hope you are not currently in a place where you feel as though you have to accept treatment that breaks your heart. I read a statement a long time ago from the book *It's Called a Breakup Because It's Broken* that resonated with me about the description of a broken heart: "Being brokenhearted is like having broken ribs. On the outside it looks like nothing's wrong, but every breath hurts."[24] Those sorts of pains get buried deep into ourselves and we often turn inward and decide that we ourselves are broken.

It's not easy to heal from those wounds, and many carry those scars and pains well past the expiration date of healthy. I refer to a story in my last book about working on a woman who was in her sixties and held a pain behind her shoulder blade (betrayal is the emotion pattern stored in that area). When we got to it through energy work, she realized the pain was from high school when her boyfriend cheated on her with her friend. Once she remembered it and released it, we both heard an audible *pop!* as the energy left her body. If you don't learn how to process through and let go of those old wounds endured during difficult relationships, they will park in the body for life. Once we learn

---

24. Greg Behrendt, Amiira Ruotola-Behrendt, *It's Called a Breakup Because It's Broken* (New York: Broadway Books, 2006), 6.

to acknowledge the pain, feel it once more and then snap and break it out of its place in the body, we can reclaim our lives.

If you are in a relationship that you are unsure of, please know that if children enter the picture, anything that bothers you now will become a much larger issue. You deserve to have a healthy, happy, loving relationship. You also need to focus on becoming the partner in a relationship that you keep hoping to find. Coming into any new relationship with the same sour behaviors that created unhealthy connections in the past will only continue to build unhealthy foundations. If you want something new, you have to do the work, and it begins with owning up to the part you play in how things progress. If you don't call yourself out on things and apologize, don't expect anyone else to do the same. Relationships hold up the mirror so that you can see yourself more clearly. Clean that mirror up.

You are powerful beyond your imagination, and what you deserve is related to exactly who you are and what you put out into the world. Ideally, you would look for a partner who is already whole, who has done the work required to be with someone like you (provided you too have done your work). No partner is here to make you whole, and that was never the goal. Finding love that complements who you are and the direction your life is heading is incredible, and I wish that for you. There is such a sense of peace and confidence when you find someone who supports all that you are. I want partners on both sides to respect each other and be inspired by each other. Each person is responsible to rise to be the best person they can possibly be. But for it to work and last, both must be in agreement on the same goal. If the goal is to be together for life, then both people need to focus on staying together. There is no room for wandering eyes or hands if you are in a committed relationship. If you have to make excuses for your partner, you might want to reconsider the deal you've struck with them. If you want to be healthy in relationships, be clear with your intentions and expectations and stick to them. Boundaries are your friends.

It is in partner relationships where we get the most out of our emotional state—good or bad. This is where the big learning lessons come in. If you are in a relationship that doesn't make your life better or you find yourself feeling less than wonderful, it might be time to really take stock in where you are currently. Remember also that there is so much power in being single. Being alone and being lonely are two very different things. You deserve to be happy and live an incredible life. If you feel like someone is holding you back, you must be willing to take responsibility for the fact that the actual person holding you back is you. Do not stay someplace that is not consistent with the level of love and affection that you are willing to give. When we line up with a partner who sucks the life from us, our emotional bodies take a beating for it. We've all been in relationships like that at some point or another, but I hope we have grown from that place and now settle for nothing less than real happiness.

The amount of people who are secretly miserable but look like they're in the best relationship in the world on social media is much higher than you may think. One day everything is fine, and the next they change their status from *married* to *divorced, in a relationship* to *single*, or the dreaded *it's complicated*. While it may be tempting to reach out, do your best not to air all your relationship problems on social media. Clean up your love space in private. Especially if you are going through a divorce, be smart and put nothing out there that can be used against you in a court of law.

My offering to you with regard to a loving relationship is this: you deserve to be happy, healthy, and loved. You must also be willing to be a partner who is happy, healthy, and loving. You will get what you put out into the world, so focus on yourself and make your life the best it can be. You cannot ask for an incredible partner if you are not one yourself. Do the work to be what you are looking for in a partner and remember: you are already whole. You are beautiful, sexy, and an amazing lover, so don't give that stuff away too freely. Everyone wants what you've got. Be choosy and hold everyone (including yourself) to the highest standards. Above all, always choose *you* when it comes to love. Fall in love with you first.

⌘ Practice: Paper Plate Magic

If you are looking for love and haven't found it yet, the practice that appears here helped me find the love of my life. I offered this little tidbit to a friend who did the same thing, and she found her love too, so maybe there is something to this! If you are already happily in love, you can use this same trick to manifest something else that you desire because it works in the same way. I have no idea why the paper plate works better than writing on plain paper, but for this exercise, it just does. Maybe it's because the paper is a circle and thus has no end, which is potentially what you are seeking in your love relationship. Maybe it's also because a plate signifies an offering. Or maybe it's because we use a plate to feed our bodies and nourish our souls, or it's the combination of being round and feeding our desire. Regardless, take out a paper plate and write every single dream you have of what you want either in a partner or in something else you strongly desire. Fill that plate and don't worry about going around the circle—it can be messy. Do not worry about the organizing of your thoughts and how they lay out. Just lay them out exactly as you are feeling them. Write down every quality you are looking for. Be extremely specific. Bring them to life with what you are writing on that plate. Don't leave out anything.

Once you've written your dream person or goal into real life, take that plate and go outside under the moon and stars and just sit with it. Feel the mindset you have created and the space for energy you are opening for this person to make their way to you. Keep that plate close to you. Put it somewhere in your house that reminds you that this is now happening. It worked for me, it worked for my friend, and I have total faith that it can work for you too! Fill your plate well.

The Stories We Tell

One way to tell whether the approaches we've taken to heal our emotions are working is noticing what stories we are telling ourselves and others. Are we still sticking to the victim story we tell everyone when they want to try to understand us? Or has it shifted so that while it is still part of our story, it is no longer the main story we tell, nor does it define us the way it used to. We don't have the same attachment to it we once did. We now clear patterns and allow ourselves to heal through it. Changing our story requires effort and awareness to omit the things we are so used to sharing. It is equally difficult to add the things we are so used to omitting.

Remember the saying that the best revenge is living well? It's totally true, but there is more to it than that—it's also getting to that power place where we are not only living well but are also no longer needing to prove to anyone just how well we are living. When we reach a new place of contentment and inner peace, we shed the compulsion to try to convince anyone otherwise. If you were a victim to a traumatic event, notice whether the dialogue surrounding the events has changed at all. See if you still carry the same resentment, attachment, or addiction to talking about it. If it hasn't left your point of conversation, don't be too hard on yourself; shifts of this kind take a lot of time and attention to make them stick. Keep working at it. You will find that it's been a really long time since you've worried yourself with that person or situation. This is a particularly big one to reveal if you are in transition from the old dialogue to the new. Pay close attention, but don't use it as the only indication that you are doing your work and putting yourself at the front for a change. After moving past the story we tell about attachments, pains, and trauma, let's get into the story we are telling ourselves about what we really want moving forward. It's just as easy to get stuck in a dialogue that may or may not be in alignment with who you are becoming. You are in charge of you.

Chapter 8
The Somatic Emotions

Let's now explore what I know best: the soft tissue and skeletal muscle system in connection to emotion. I believe there are basic life experiences that occur that we may or may not choose to store and remember. If it was just a simple experience, it won't likely have any effect on the body. If, however, an experience was a significant traumatic or joyful event, it's likely the body memory will be involved.

When it comes to the distinction between tissue memory, cellular memory, and muscle memory, I do not believe these to be the same: cellular memory is carried within the cells themselves, and tissue memory can live in both muscle and fascia, *but* these do not hold memory in the same way (although they do work in tandem). It's been proven that muscles have their own memory of movement and holding experiences similar to the way the mind remembers. I liken the muscles to the mind's second-in-command when it comes to storage and holding patterns. Fascia is how the memories move and can be released. In a nutshell, everything is closely interlinked but no single component is identical to the other two. For the purpose of this section, we will refer to everything under the general label of body memory or the more accurate term, somatic memory (*somatic* being the fancy term for the body).

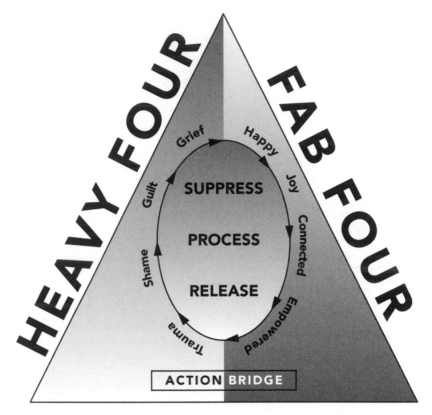

Figure 3: Somatic Emotion Chart

The most prominent emotion experiences stored within the body tissues are trauma, shame, guilt, and grief. Each are followed by a bridge of action behaviors that, when experienced, can bring a person from the suppression of an emotion into the act of processing and releasing the old pains associated with the original emotional trauma. These action behaviors are suppression, process, and release. If you suppress emotion, then the emotions of the original trauma become the ones that will remain. As I see it, suppression of emotions is still an action you are taking in order to avoid facing it and shifting it. If, however, you choose to go through the process to release (the opposite action to suppression), then you can get to the side of happiness, joy, connection, and empowerment. Happiness is something we feel and experience commonly as bliss, pleasure, and contentment. Joy is not as common as happiness and is a stronger rooted emotion experienced through the body in terms of true release and connectedness within oneself. And connection refers to a positive feeling expressed along with balance within the whole system. Nothing is disconnected; it's an action of acceptance. Empowerment is a place of not only being joyful and connected but also a sense of groundedness and rootedness in the balance and peacefulness that are now exuding from within. At this level, confidence enters your life that can be better felt than explained.

The Heavy Side of Body Emotions: The Painful Four

Trauma

Trauma may not be an emotion that you can chart, but when it comes to the emotional layer of the body, it is one of the top emotional patterns that we must treat in order to heal. Trauma sets in at the moment of impact. It can be something that occurred physically resulting in an actual wound, or it can be something emotionally scarring that lands the wound deeply into the layers of the body. The term *trauma* in relation to the body can refer to every single thing that has affected the body in a negative way; it's something that has happened to you without your permission. Post-traumatic stress disorder (PTSD) is primarily regarded as a mental disorder that appears as the result of an incredibly disturbing and painful event that a person is not able to bypass and live freely beyond. Many veterans suffer from PTSD, as does anyone who experienced something that shocked their systems into a new circuit. I was diagnosed with PTSD as a result of losing my father so unexpectedly. The psychiatrist I saw told me he believed that while I had done extraordinary work to help cope with the shock and loss of my beloved father, I was still living in a state of PTSD all these years later. PTSD doesn't just settle itself into our minds and affect the way we behave; it also changes the dynamics of our bodies and how we handle and process life events from that point forward.

Shame

Shame is explained in a number of ways, but I understand it through my point of reference, the body. When we think of the concept of shame, we may think of actions intended to humiliate, mortify, embarrass, or punish. The way our minds perceive shame and our bodies store those perceptions cut deep and hard. Shame is a terribly difficult emotion for people to explore due to their complete disdain of the experience and the scars left afterward. Shame is one of the deadliest of the body sins because it is nearly impossible to get our minds to change the dialogue that started the feelings in the first place. It is difficult in large part because whatever the dialogue was came from outside of us. It was thrown at us and then anchored down as a part of our natural talk cycle. It lives so deep in our psyche that we barely remember anything before it set in. Someone who has felt deeply shamed in their lives tends to carry the belief of not feeling worthy of anything good, and their sense of self-loathing and punishment go on and on. The tissues hold such loathing that they almost feel as if they have stiffened when connecting to it either energetically or physically. I've found when working with shame that we get more results when people can get to the self-talk of "I can't change the past," and into "I can only focus on the present moment and in this moment, I forgive myself" instead. Shame tends not to pair with a forgiveness of anyone but ourselves because shame is something we take in as something we did was wrong. It's a self-punishment and it's very hard to stop punishing ourselves. The person who created the first deep wound is long gone, yet we continue and turn their words into self-deprecation. Again, shame is all about "me," rooted in painful feelings regarding how we feel about ourselves. I firmly believe that the original cause comes from outside ourselves but when those feelings settle into the body, they turn into shame.

Guilt

Guilt and shame are best friends of the very worst kind. Guilt is something that many people have used to get us to comply. If shame is punishment of who you are, guilt is what keeps you down because it weighs a ton. Guilt and shame together tell you that you are wrong or less than, never good enough, pretty enough, smart enough, creative enough, anything and everything "enough." While shame makes the tissues cry in our bodies, guilt hardens those tissues. In my opinion, guilt is easier to work with than shame for hands-on work, but both really suck the life force out of us. And if there is shame, there is sure to be guilt nearby. The self-talk with these two are interchangeable. Guilt can often be more about the awareness that actions caused someone else pain. Guilt is something we consider having done wrong, which means that even if what was done wasn't based in reality, it's an action. It's also a very powerful tool to use to get someone to do what you want them to do. A parent notoriously guilts their children into doing what they want not realizing that the guilt continues long after they completed the task asked of them. If I were sick and stayed home from school or missed work, I felt it necessary to continue to berate myself and feel guilty for the entire time I had stepped out on my commitment. Guilt is heavy, hardens in the body, and can easily become a highly repetitive process within the self. Do your best to become aware of your own guilt behaviors, and do your best to lighten up that sort of inner dialogue.

Grief

While everyone feels sad from time to time, grief is different—much more lasting. Grief is something likened to having children. People who have children tell you that you can't possibly understand what it's like because you don't have children of your own. People who don't have children find this statement offensive because they *do* know love. They may love their pets like their own children and find the notion condescending. To be fair, it can sound dismissive, almost as if we are disregarding the person without children's capacity and depth for love. However, unless you actually do have children, there is a bit of truth to it! Those who don't have a life that revolves around children don't fully understand life with them. That doesn't mean they can't *appreciate* or *understand* it on a conceptual level, but appreciation, understanding, and experience are not the same. There are details and nuance to life with kids: for example, you can't leave babies at home like you can a pet while you leave the house to run errands. Every single moment of the day needs to be accounted for, and someone must be with young children at all times to keep them safe. There is obviously more, but I'm using this example to make the analogy. It's the same with grief. When you have lost something that breaks you down completely, people can sympathize and appreciate, but your grief doesn't live with *them* day in and day out like it does with you. You can't adequately explain grief because it goes so much deeper than description. Grieving is extremely personal, and no one has the right to tell you how to grieve or for how long. The loss never really goes away, and the grief never really leaves you; it just figures out a way to live with you and you figure out a way to keep it tucked in your front pocket or worn over your shoulder. You eventually learn to move forward in your life with the new stowaway always present. Within the body's tissues, grief can drop an anchor that changes the dynamics of how you move in every way from that point forward. Once grief has planted itself in our lives, we begin living a two-dimensional parallel life. The one that is the current reality we are in, and the one that could have been had the loss not occurred. With the loss of someone we deeply love and cherish, we may move forward but there is always that little part that keeps time. How old would they be now, how different would our life be if they were still in it, what choices would be different, and what would I have made of myself if I hadn't fallen into such deep grief and despair—all these things come up more often than we may like to admit. Time does not heal all wounds where grief is concerned.

Grief is the emotional component most likely to be coupled with serious disease. It's considered acceptable if a person dies of a broken heart, but when we couple the emotional grief with illness such as cancers, there are varied levels of acceptance. Grief does not necessarily cause cancer, but there is also a lot of speculation that many autoimmune diseases (such as inflammation) are deeply rooted in the trauma/shame/guilt/grief emotion cycle.

If you keep any of these negative experiences suppressed inside the body and are unwilling to talk or even think about them with the intention of release, they can fester and turn into something really dangerous to the whole system. It is not until we learn how to process our experience and release their roots that we will able to experience a freedom that results in healing. This does not mean that the experience is suddenly erased from your memory. It means that your attachment to it is no longer the same. It becomes less and less the story we tell when we choose to identify ourselves in our history. We think of it less. We tell it less. We aren't attached to it in the same way, and finally, it simply loses its hold on us. This is forgiveness in action. This is exactly the behavior that my friend and spiritual counselor Ashli Callaway defined as "forgiveness as an action." She says:

> For me, forgiveness is the practice of remembering a painful event, accepting that it happened as it did, and letting go of my attachments to it and the pain it caused. It is not forgetting, condoning, tolerating, enabling or self-sacrificing. It is accepting and letting go. It is an act of self-love.

This is the practice that will take you over the bridge and directly into life with the fabulous four (more on that in the next section). You deserve to live your life from this space. I have supreme faith in your healing and your ability to live your very best life. And that life begins as soon as you make it your intention and follow it all the way through.

⌘ Practice: Forgiveness Seven Times for Seven Days

The thing about forgiveness that I think we often miss is that it is about forgiving the part of ourselves that has the attachment to the person or situation that caused us pain. It's not about forgiving that person. Many times, they don't care if we do or don't anyway. The power lies in forgiving ourselves for the part we played in any of it and severing the ties that kept us bound to whatever the situation was (in the section on energy we will discuss cord cutting). This practice is about forgiving ourselves.

For seven days in a row, be willing to do this practice. To forgive ourselves, we must be willing to really look at ourselves in the mirror. For seven days, we look at ourselves in the mirror and repeat the words: "I forgive myself." We repeat these words seven times in a row. Keep a sheet of paper near you and mark off each affirmation. Over the course of the seven days, the way you are able to see yourself will change. I did this exercise at my lowest point, and it changed me—it is a very powerful exercise. I highly encourage you to do this exercise and go back to it whenever you need to get back in balance with yourself.

The Practice of Flooding

There is a term I learned in my yoga training, *samskara*, which translates to "mind grooves." It is the mental patterns that have been repeated so many times that they carve out actual thought grooves. Imagine a rake being pulled in the sand repeatedly in only one pattern. The pattern would only be able to look like the number of lines of the rake tines—no squiggles or circles, just the straight lines of the rake always from the same starting point to the same end point without deviation.

When we attempt to change the dialogue in our mind, we must create different grooves that overlap or cancel out the preexisting ones already in place. If we decide to try a different tool, for example, a smaller rake, but still go in the same direction, we will have little luck getting any meaningful changes to occur. When taking the approach to change, we must change the ingrained patterns that play on the soundtrack in our heads. We must do so with such force that we flood the whole sound system to play another tune. Imagine taking a giant bucket of water and pouring it over the lines we have raked. If we flood it, we can change the lines' placement and start over with a new tool on a fresh canvas. So it goes with the thoughts in our head and the way in which we talk to ourselves. We have to flood the system if we want it to create new tracks. We must consistently show up and speak to our whole body as if what we say really matters—because it does! Flooding the internal system with positive affirmative dialogue can actually transform us on a cellular level. Positive talk can help recreate the internal system into a stronger, suppler version of yourself inside and out. If you let it, this small but powerful task can rearrange your entire system from the inside out.

If you are familiar with the work of Dr. Masaru Emoto in his book *The Secret Life of Water,* then you know he did many studies to show that the consciousness of the human mind had a great impact on the molecular structure of water.[25] He tested the crystallization of water after saying both positive and negative affirmations to the water. The positive affirmations changed the vibrational makeup of the water. Something that was originally chlorinated and could not produce crystals under the microscope, was transformed to being able to produce them after he had five hundred people say "thank you" to the water. It is not just his work that explores the idea that a person's dialogue and thoughts set out a vibrational frequency that can affect health in a most powerful way. Thoughts become reality. The way in which you speak to yourself inside your mind can propel you to better health or to a total collapse. It's always your choice.

⌘ Practice: Flood Your System with Kindness

First thing in the morning, think or say aloud the words *thank you* and see how much it changes the start of your day. If you think that only water can change with those sweet, simple words, you're in for a surprise. You can transform a great deal by starting each and every morning with *thank you*. Be grateful for the small things. When you get in the shower and wash your body, give love to it and compliment it. Remove the inner hurtful dialogue that you may be used to. Change your inner dialogue. An affirmation cycle for one week would be:

25. Dr. Masaru Emoto, *The Secret Life of Water* (Hillsboro, OR: Beyond Words Publishing 2005).

1. Every cell in my body is operating at healthy, optimum levels.
2. I love my body exactly as it is.
3. I am healthy and vibrant.
4. The DNA in my body corrects and restores itself now.
5. Today, I am grateful for every part of my life.
6. I am surrounded by love.
7. Any parts of me that are out of balance correct themselves now.

⌘ Practice: Mirror Work to Balance the Duality Within

Quite frequently, the reflection in the mirror seems to be the opposite of what you feel inside, almost like you're looking at another world. Your reflection is the other half of the current reality you are standing in. When I was super anxious, I was always surprised at how in control I looked in the mirror.

This is a practice that sounds simple but is powerful work. When you are scared, sad, angry, off balance, nervous, etc., go into the bathroom and look at yourself in the mirror. Touch the part of your reflection that feels most out of balance. If it's your emotional space, touch your reflection in the mirror's head or somewhere on your reflection's face. If it's your heart space and you are feeling sad or heartbroken, touch your reflection's heart. Do not touch your own physical body—touch the person in the mirror's body. Do not lose eye contact with this practice. Look yourself in the eye, touch the part of you that needs the opposite energy in the reflection of the mirror. Again, be sure you are physically touching the mirror. Notice how quickly this helps offset the original feelings. This is how you can gain strength and power from your own dual self.

The Action Bridge of Body Emotions

There are behaviors you can put in place that can either keep you stuck where you are (where the emotions are not processed or released), or that can elevate you to an entirely new existence (the successful processing and release of the initial traumas). These behaviors are more or less either ones that bring you over the hump or keep you under it.

As mentioned earlier in the section on EMDR research, at the moment any trauma is inflicted, it freezes in time. Our job is to work with the initial trauma and help it to step out of the past and be processed in a way that makes it livable inside yourself. Look for a way to let the memories advance in maturity (from the time of the trauma) so that you can see them through your current eyes. Doing so can reshape those memories to the point where they no longer take root and replay your old story of anguish. Here is where the painful story you tell changes and loses its strength. In this space, you find freedom.

Suppression

If you are unwilling to experience and release emotions, you will eventually create physical upset within yourself. Suppression is one of the most toxic behaviors we can fall into. We don't like to express when we are angry, sad, fearful, remorseful, or powerless. We like to maintain control or the appearance of being in control to the point that it backfires on us. All of this pressure will turn inward to fester and explode. Heart issues, high blood pressure, and stroke all correlate emotionally to not expressing feelings of anger, aggravation, and confusion in a healthy way. Instead of being expressed and released, they block the pathway of emotion in the energy body. The shortened breath of experiencing an emotion response that we are not willing to share can physically block the blood flow, which is a dangerous pattern. We don't have to yell and scream when we feel something unpleasant, but we do need to be more willing to share how we are feeling and clear the space from which it came.

Process

The actions we take to find peace with our unresolved emotions is the work of the process. In order to release the traumas, we must go through the work of remembering a wound, locating the attachment of that experience to the parts of our bodies that are storing that experience, and pull it out of its frozen place to the now and deal with it. The action of processing in order to release is no small task. It will require a lot of effort on your part to get there.

Release

The action that leads to empowerment is release. To release within the body can be likened to renouncing a physical habit or mental patterns. It is letting go of something really heavy from life to the point that there is no longer any attachment to whatever it *was*. It is freeing to no longer have any attachment to whatever plagued us. Release doesn't mean it erases itself from your mind, but it does change the way it has been dialogued within. That is where the magic lives. Release allows us the lightness and clarity with which to enter a new phase of life. It is understanding what happened from an objective point of view and really seeing how we chose to store it within our body's tissues. Release requires facing the past head on, processing events as they occurred, and letting go of the attachments to the experience. It then becomes true liberation through which feelings of bliss can enter freely and work their magic of healing and recovering.

The Positive Side of Body Emotions: The Fab Four

Happiness

Happiness is a feeling we experience as one of the lightest and most glorious emotions possible. Though extremely close in experience to joy, happiness is lighter and experienced more often than joy, which is deeper and more lasting. Happiness is associated with pleasure, lightness, laughter, and feelings of bliss. Feeling this way is something we experience while on the way to the deeper tissue layers that can store joy.

Joy

Joy is the foundation and fountain of youth for a healthy body and mind. Happiness and bliss merged into a single emotion, joy is something the whole body can experience while simultaneously anchoring down into itself. Trauma is not the only experience that can make a home in your body—when we experience joy, it can lock into the muscle and tissues because it is strong enough to be retrieved from muscle memory to bring increased health and harmony to the body. When a person experiences joy, every cell and tissue locks it in and remembers it. The experience of true joy is something we can tap into from within the tissues to help in healing other body layers. Joy is a blessing to behold; the next time you find yourself belly laughing, loving, or simply accepting yourself without reservations, judgment, or fear, hold on tight and remember it well! As far as body experiences are concerned, joy and bliss can easily be interchanged, but joy gives you an open spine, and a little extra lift.

Connection

Being connected is much like being centered. You feel a link within yourself that radiates out into the world with others. The feeling of connection allows cells to move without obstruction, blood and plasma to flow well, and the lungs to expand and take in full breaths. The energy body and the emotional state of the body are both balanced. Connectedness is a state of mind and a comfort in the whole body that occurs when a person is rooted and present with themselves. In this place, we are not trying to run away from anything we are holding or hiding. It is a sense of feeling safe and at peace within one's self. This feeling usually happens when a person has released other body emotions, thus allowing the experience of true openness. Connectedness is a glorious experience; hopefully once you have it, you can set the daily intention to manage to operate life from that space. Once you've felt this in your body, it will become a priority to live from feeling connected. You will become astutely aware when you get out of balance and will be much better equipped to remedy it quickly.

Empowerment

Being empowered is being rooted, grounded, strong, supple, and healthy, mixed with a sense of trust in yourself and the world. It is a freedom, but not a flighty kind of freedom. It is a power place that connects you into the whole world through your body, a feeling of being centered but with more strength and stamina. Empowerment is a place of connection to all your body parts and the physical and cosmic world that surrounds you. It is a place to experience your strongest and mightiest self safely. To be empowered implies the ability to feel every experience without strong attachment but also never avoiding or pretending a situation is not anything but exactly what it is. Though a place of considerable power and fierce energy, it is mellowed out in a way that it doesn't carry any friction. In a body experiencing empowerment, the tissues are soft and supple, and muscles are more pliable to the touch. Even a muscular person you'd assume would be difficult to work with is not because the empowered body holds a depth of understanding and power. People who experience empowerment have generally already had some sort of breakthrough or emotional release that allowed them to release pain, trauma, shame, guilt, and/or sorrow in a way they may not have in their past. They are free and you can feel it. I want this feeling for all of us; it is a beautiful and strong place from which we can all operate.

You have the power within you to experience every single one of these somatic emotions, from the heaviest to the lightest and most vibrant body memory you've ever experienced. We just need to learn how to change the dialogue and awareness of the past into a place where we can live peacefully. Once we face and work with our shadow sides, they lose their darkness and the shadows disappear, just like when the sun comes out. Internal work is truly the game changer for health and healing. I know you can do it. You deserve to live with freedom from the pains inflicted upon you. Now you are wise enough to change the patterns and claim victory where you once might have felt powerless. No more. Onward and upward we go.

Part IV
The Energetic Body

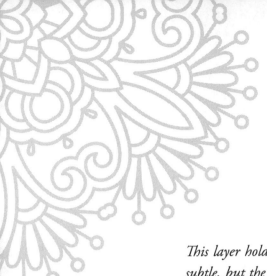

This layer holds your magic keys. The shifts on this level can be subtle, but the results are powerful. Hold on tight, dear friends, because here is where the magic comes to life if you allow yourself to believe. You can heal and you were meant to heal. You were never meant to stay down for so long. This life is a gift, and I set the intention with you to open it up and try it on. You are magic.

Chapter 9

Healthcare Practices and Therapies for the Energy Body

The energetic layer or subtle layer of the body is often overlooked as its own complete aspect of the body. Oftentimes woven into the spiritual or emotional treatments without recognizing its own part to play. In Western culture, the energy body is not considered part of the original trinity—body, mind, and spirit—except in some cases when it is lumped in with spirit. Energy lives inside us and all around us, but external energy is different from the energy inside our bodies. For the purpose of body healing, we will focus on the energy living within our bodies that, when treated, can balance our bodies in incredible ways. I believe this is the layer that holds the magic keys to full healing. Without this piece, we are missing a great opportunity to clear and balance a part of the body that is so subtle but so powerful. This is where the terms *chi* (or *qi*), *ki*, and *prana* were created. The Chinese *chi,* Japanese *ki,* and Vedic *prana* all refer to the same thing— the universal life force energy within each of us. In the West, researchers have created the term "scalar waves," or "scalar light" as a more clinical term that works with chi/ki/prana that peole can accept and understand more readily. Working with the chi/ki/prana is a sacred practice and can be accessed in several ways.

Energy

We've all learned that energy cannot be created or destroyed, only transferred. This goes for energy both inside yourself and outside yourself. Energy can be transmuted and made into something usable within yourself. This is the very best kind of energy transfer.

When it comes to energy and how it applies to the energetic body, there are quite a few angles we need to approach to better understand the whole. We will start with the basic definitions and then look further into each area. The energy field itself can be described in many ways. Some refer to it as a frequency or a magnetic field. Others consider it a vibration. And still others consider it to be defined by a specific temperature (heat specifically). Stephen Watson, several time world champion in Taiji Push Hands (*tui shou*) as well as a disciplined student of the Tao, explains energy in a way I can appreciate: "Energy takes form. Forms of energy get named. We feel these forms. We taste these forms. We shape these forms. We are shaped by these forms. There may be one energy and infinite forms. There may be some manageable number of categories of these forms. It is of no matter; the energy is energy."

The Energy Connection to Health

Before the Western medical approach replaced traditional thinking, healing practices in every culture around the world assessed the quality and strength of the energy flow in and around a person to aid in diagnosing their health; it was not considered taboo or strange. Then Western thinking and practice spread, separating the body from the mind and removing the energy component completely. While the West has given us amazing technology and cutting-edge treatments that save many lives, forgetting or discounting the original practices that include our vital energy for whole body healing is a huge mistake. Now considered alternative medicine, energy medicine is really the medicine of the ages. And what's more, scientists and research are proving that these beliefs were right all along. Nobel Prize–winning biochemist Albert Szent-Gyorgyi said, "In every culture and in every medical tradition before ours, healing was accomplished by moving energy."[26]

Foundations for Energy Cultivation

Practices such as Traditional Chinese Medicine and exercise practices such as tai chi and qi gong work with the movements and ideas that our internal energy is running along the meridian channels exactly the way water runs through a hose. Should something become obstructed, it's as if we bent the hose and the energy gets stagnated. If a certain area is

---

26. Albert Szent-Gyorgyi, "Energy Psychology," Ephemeral Energy. https://www.ephemeralenergy.com/treatments/energy-psychology/.

blocked, it can result in physical illness and blocks in the emotional and energetic body. In this chapter we cover tai chi, qi gong, yoga, meditations, and affirmations, as well as visualizations. Working with the energy body is a big key to healing; without it, whole body healing is nearly impossible.

✿ Practice: Feel Body Energy

Begin by rubbing your hands together until you feel heat. Look at your hands after you've created the heat and notice if there is redness, or small white spotty or blotchy areas in the palms. These indicators let you know that your energy channels have opened. To feel the energy, start with your hands almost touching. Bring your open palms so close that you can feel heat or static between the hands. Imagine there is an energy ball between your two palms. Bring your hands further apart until you no longer feel the energy. Move them back toward each other and feel the energy again. Now, don't move the hands beyond the sphere of being able to feel the heat, static, vibration, or energy. Play with your energy ball for just a minute. Move your hands in different angles still holding on to that energy ball. Close your eyes and continue to play with that ball. Notice if the feeling becomes easier to feel with eyes open or closed.

Where did that energy come from? Is it from the heat you created between your hands when you rubbed them? Where did the energy come from that created the heat through the energy channels? It came from inside you! You have a constant flow of energy at all times inside your body, and that energy is your essence, which keeps your body running smoothly.

We consider energy to be physical because it is inside the body, but it also lives out beyond the parameters of physical skin and bone structure. It can be seen, felt, touched, and understood, but not on a physical level. It runs through you in every way. It lives in each breath you take. It lives in your physical movements. It lives in your emotional and spiritual bodies as well. It is your driving force of vitality. It lives inside your blood, tissue, and plasma, and along the matrix of the fascia that encases every muscle and organ in your body. It lives outside your body and makes up what is known as your aura. Your energy makes up your primary essence.

Medical and Physical Practices from China

There are several parts under the Traditional Chinese Medicine (TCM) label you will see spread out in the sections to follow in this chapter. TCM includes acupuncture (with needles), acupressure and tui na (massage), tai chi and qi gong practice (exercise), herbal medicine, and nutrition consultation (diet). Traditional Chinese Medicine works with the body's chi or life force energy. The manner in which chi moves through the channels within the body, as well as the quality and strength of the energy flow, can help determine whether someone is healthy or compromised. According to which channels are weak or blocked relate to what specific organ system will be treated.

In Chinese Medicine, the meridian pathways come in one pair of twelve channels each. In 1960, North Korean surgeon and researcher Dr. Bong Han Kim was able to prove the existence of meridian channels. He reported them to be tubular structures that existed outside of both the lymphatic and the blood vessel passageways.[27] He also saw the tubular structures on the surface of the organs below the skin. He asserted that these structures were a vital part of the cardiovascular system. In another study, scientists used a CT scan to create contrasting imaging to see and measure energy in the acupuncture points versus non-acupuncture points. Published in the *Journal of Electron Spectroscopy and Related Phenomena*, the study showed that by injecting a dye into the acupuncture points, they were able to see the line of the energy along its channel. Along non-acupuncture points, even with the dye, no lines showed up on the scans. This proved that there were "microvascular structures that clearly correspond to the map of acupuncture points."[28]

Tools Used in Traditional Chinese Medicine (TCM)

A person classically trained in Traditional Chinese Medicine will know how to make herbal formulas and teas specifically for their patients. If they do not dispense the herbs

---

27. Craig Lewis, "Korean Researchers Claim Scientific Evidence of Meridians," BuddhistDoor.net, May 6, 2016, https://www.buddhistdoor.net/news/korean-researchers-claim-scientific-evidence-of-meridians.

28. Azriel ReShel, "Scientific Research Finally Proved That Meridians Exist," CODE, January 25, 2018, https://www.lifecoachcode.com/2018/01/25/scientific-research-proved-meridians-exist/.

themselves as a loose herbal mixture to make tea with, they will certainly have premixed herb bottles that usually consist of little pellets or in tea form.[29] Do not confuse acupuncture in any way with dry needling as it is not even remotely the same thing. Dry needling is used for muscles and to pop the lactic acid out of trigger points. Physical therapists and some chiropractors or naturopaths primarily use dry needling. A true classical acupuncturist is licensed to practice Chinese Medicine. Be sure that you separate those modalities completely in your mind. The only thing those two have in common is the acupuncture needles.

Other things a classically trained TCM practitioner may offer as a service include cupping (not the new trendy cupping for muscles, but the original cupping with several glass bowls that are heated and used to suction out excess elemental wind from the lungs). Cupping is magnificent as a treatment with needles and herbs to help with any respiratory condition among other things.

Moxibustion (moxa) is another tool specific to TCM. Moxibustion uses mugwort either as a cone placed directly on the skin to burn near the meridian channel the needle is stimulating, or as a stick that is indirectly burned near the area but held by the practitioner. Moxa is used when a person has a cold or a cold condition, meaning that energy is stagnant in a certain area. Moxa is used to warm the meridians and help disperse the stagnation. Moxibustion can be used to increase blood circulation and help with the pelvic area, the uterus, and to stimulate menstruation. It has also long been used to help turn breech babies. In order to use moxibustion, a person must have an acupuncture license.

If you are seeing a TCM practitioner, they will also discuss nutrition as therapy. There are no "forbidden" foods per se, but they instead offer a better food profile that will benefit your specific health and energy profile. The recommendations are the result of the belief that a balanced diet includes five flavors or tastes: (1) spicy to warm, (2) sour to cool, (3) bitter to cool, (4) sweet to strengthen, and (5) salty to cool. For a nutrition consultation, you might be asked to bring a food journal to your sessions. The practitioner will also analyze your tongue to look for color coating, whether the sides are scalloped, dryness, and cracks on the surface. Each of these points give the practitioner insight into the health of the organs throughout the body.

---

29. David Cosio, Erica H. Lin, "6 Traditional Chinese Medicine Techniques" PPM.com, August 15, 2015, https://www.practicalpainmanagement.com/patient/treatments/alternative/6-traditional-chinese-medicine-techniques.

A Chinese medical practitioner will do a pulse diagnosis at the start of each session in order to listen to the six different pulse points on the inside of your wrists. What we in America might use to take a pulse count, a TCM practitioner places three fingers vertically along as there are three light sounds and three deeper sounds to listen for on each inner wrist. This is somewhat of an art form among those who practice pulse diagnosis. The first category is the rate of the pulse, which may be fast or slow. This pulse shows up if there is a fever or inflammation. A slow pulse might indicate a cold, or stagnant or sluggish chi in the body. Next is the pulse's strength. A strong pulse indicates too much of something or an excess of some kind, such as high blood pressure, excessive anger, or too much stress. A weak pulse shows the opposite: deficiency, weakness, lack of sleep, low blood pressure, and possible depression. Next they feel for the pulse's width. Here they listen for a thin or thready pulse, which would indicate nutrition deficiencies, weakness, exhaustion, poor digestion, or insomnia. Its opposite, a slippery or rolling pulse, might indicate excess phlegm, a backed-up digestive system, sinus problems, or allergies.[30]

Going even deeper (for each pair of meridians it's three soft and three deeper to gain access to all organs) are the pulse positions and what they tell. On the left wrist, the practitioner listens for the heart and small intestine, the liver and gallbladder, and the kidney and bladder. On the right wrist they listen for lung and large intestine, spleen and stomach, and pericardium and triple burner (both are organ systems in Chinese Medicine for which there is no perfect Western correspondence).

The meridians are energy lines that flow along the matrix of the fascia in the body. Each meridian is a channel that governs a specific organ in the body. According to Chinese Medicine, the organs all have high and low emotions that correspond to that organ's actual function. Each organ also corresponds to cravings of food types and times of day where they are strongest and weakest. There are twelve primary paired meridians and two single meridian channels (one conception vessel considered yin/feminine and one governing vessel considered yang/masculine that run midline). Six of the primary pairs are considered yin/feminine and run up the body. The other six are yang/masculine and flow down the body. Each meridian has an organ and an element relating to it as well as a corresponding emotion.

---

30. Nadia Bouhdili, "How Pulse Diagnosis Works" (October 8, 2015). https://www.dc-acupuncture.com/physical -health/how-pulse-diagnosis-works

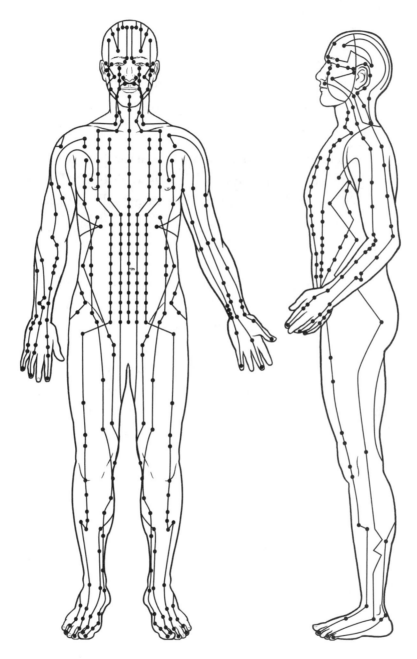

Figure 4: Meridian Channels

Yin	Yang	Imbalanced Emotion
liver	gallbladder	anger, frustration
pericardium	triple burner	fight, flight, freeze response
kidney	bladder	fear
lung	large intestine	grief, depression
spleen	stomach	worry, anxiety
heart	small intestine	hatred, impatience

Energy becomes balanced when treated. If you are able to feel your own body energy, you might feel a strange momentum of energy around your whole being. The energy may circle around your whole body with ease and flow. The energy will be balanced, vibrant, open, and offer a happier feeling.

Tai Chi

Tai chi (or taiji) is a martial arts practice. Although a slow-moving style focused on the health benefits of relaxation, breath control, and allowing energy to guide movements, it is still a martial arts practice with specific applications attached. Tai chi is a deceptive form of internal martial arts where practitioners aim to use an opponent's energy against themselves. There are several forms and styles of tai chi practices, but all can serve as a healing practice that strengthens the bones all the way down to the marrow. It is a wonderful practice for people of any age and condition. A focus on applying the martial arts aspects such as posture, specific footing, and body movements is an important part of this practice.

Qi Gong

In the West, we often interchange the terms and practices of tai chi and qi gong (or chi kung) because the movements are slow and similar, but qi gong has a different focus not on the martial arts applications but on the energy moving within the body and the use of the breath to help guide that energy through any blocks within the channels. It is a health-focused approach rather than a martial arts-focused approach. Qi gong is a light practice that is incredibly healing and beneficial for everyone no matter their age or condition.

❋ PRACTICE: CULTIVATE HEART SPACE ENERGY

I teamed up with many time world champion martial artist and friend Stephen Watson to offer this simple loving exercise. There are only two things to remember here: gentle and soft, and heart space—the space between heaven and earth.

Stand upright barefoot upon the earth. Allow the earth energy to be felt through the feet. As you stand, round your shoulders slightly, soften the knees, and imagine your tailbone as a long tail that acts as the third balance point along with your feet. Breathe from the belly. Inhale, and allow the belly to quietly expand out like a balloon being blown up. Exhale, and feel the belly return easily in toward the navel. Feel your heart space energetically. There is no pressure in your body. Mix heaven and earth through your body and through your breath. Bring the hands up toward your heart space on the inhale, and exhale bring the hands back down to your sides. Inhale and bring the energy into your heart space, bringing your hands only as high as the heart itself as the palms arrive just beneath the area you feel your heart's presence to be … they are not quite at the heart but beneath, supportive of the heart just as the heart itself is supportive of all in nature. Exhale and lower the hands down to the sides. There is no pressure. It's almost bouncy, but it's not.

Rhythmically returning, the legs receive the settling body and the Being that settles with it … you. It's rooted deeply into the earth with the legs and feet and rooted high in the sky with the hips up to the head. Incorporating the breath into the movement helps with cultivating the energy into the heart on the inhale as well as release the energy through the exhale to return to the earth. You don't have to count how many times to practice this relaxing, loving movement. It's about inviting the energy into yourself through the breath, through the openness of the mind.

(To see this practice in its entirety of Mixing Heaven and Earth as a nei gong practice, see Stephen Watson: Cultivating HeartSpace Energy Video: Bit.ly/WholeBodyHealthHeartspaceQigong.)

Medical and Physical Practices from India

Ayurveda

Ayurvedic medicine from India (*ayurveda* is a Sanskrit word meaning "the complete knowledge for long life") is a study that has more than five thousand years of practice that does not prescribe one-size-fits-all in its approach to healing. An Ayurvedic practitioner will go over every detail they can find about the person they are treating to help them balance their system. Things an Ayurvedic practitioner checks are family history, and palpating the wrists (but in a way different from the pulse points according to Chinese Medicine), the tongue, the eyes and the nails. They will listen to the heart and lungs as well as the intestines. They will identify both the client's dosha (more on those next) and their elemental profile. They also review the organ systems, metabolic waste, and digestion concerns as well as any issues concerning tissues within the body structure.

In this system, people are categorized into three *doshas* (body types). All relate to how the energies of the five elements—space, fire, air, water, and earth—manifest in the body. All combine in various ways to govern the body's functions. Your dosha is a way of life according to diet and lifestyle for the healthiest outcome that works within your specific constitution. No one is just one dosha; among the three types, everyone relates to one dosha more than the other two. As an example: someone may be more vata/pitta dosha. Therefore, their body would be more on the airy side and the mind may be more fiery and focused. Digestion varies with what we eat, how we handle things in our lives, and the weather. We make adjustments according to where we are currently in those conditions.

1. Vata: ether/air—the combination of air and space. It governs circulation, all movement in the body, elimination, as well as movements of the mind. Anything moving is vata. These body types are long and lean.

2. Pitta: fire/water—the combination of fire and water. It governs physical as well as mental digestion. Transformation and metabolic processes in the body belong to water and fire. These body types tend to be stalky and muscular.

3. Kapha: earth/water—the heavy elements. Governs lubrication and hydration. The structure elements of the body are earth—bones, muscle, and fats. Structure, stability, and growth (among other things) are also earth related. These body types tend to be larger and move slower.

If a person is out of balance, the practitioner might prescribe simple treatments such as a shift in lifestyle, habits, and diet. If the imbalance is significant, the advice is usually a protocol known as panchakarma that might take thirty, sixty, or even ninety days.

Marma Points

Marma points on the body are the points where two or more kinds of tissues meet within the body such as muscles, veins, ligaments, joints, or bones. They are considered the body's energetic points and the place to treat and balance the body's prana. They are different from the meridian channels and acupuncture points of Chinese Medicine. Confusingly, you might find Chinese Medicine texts refer to the body's chakras and Ayurvedic texts that refer to meridians. One does not discount the other, but they do not offer the same information, with the exception that everything is in service of balancing the body's essential life force energy for health.

There are believed to be 107 or 108 marma points throughout the body, a number that varies among the research. The energy from the different marma points connect to the chakra system of the body in Ayurvedic practice. Stimulating the marma points is done with finger pressure massage movements.

The Chakras

The chakras give us another way to both understand and heal the body on a physical, emotional, energetic, and spiritual level. The chakras are your body's energy centers that negotiate both physical and subtle energies. The chakras are important with regard to the way emotions manifest through the energy body and into the physical body. Each chakra is associated with a specific area of the body, and the body has seven main chakras that store emotions. When we talk about things like a broken heart, we know instinctively that we are talking about the heart chakra, the energetic heart—not the actual organ. We have always known the heart as two specific entities—the emotional part of ourselves and a specific organ in the body with four chambers. There are actually several hundreds of chakras throughout the body, but we will focus on the seven main ones. These seven chakras govern the places of energetic consciousness, and each correlate to the energetic spine (*sashumna*), the actual spine, as well as the nerve plexus. The chakras are vital to our overall health and well-being; to dismiss this could be detrimental to both. Each chakra represents a state of consciousness and has a specific feeling and tone. Beginning at the base of the spine, we start with the following:

The first chakra, known as the root chakra, is located at the lower end of the spinal column and corresponds to the sacral plexus. The Sanskrit name for this chakra is the *muladhara;* its color is red. The sound associated with this chakra is *lam,* and its lotus has four petals. This chakra governs the connection to the earth and earthly materials, including material possessions, influence, fame, and fortune.

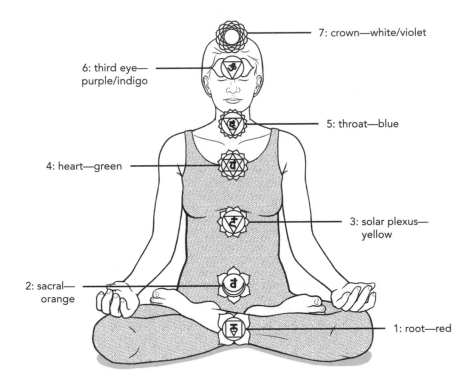

Figure 5: Chakras on the Body Seated

The second chakra, known as the sacral chakra, is located around the reproductive organs and sacrum. The Sanskrit name for this chakra is *swadhisthana,* and its color is orange. This chakra is associated with the water element, and it governs creativity and sexual energy. The sound associated with this chakra is *vam,* and its lotus has six petals.

The third chakra, known as the solar plexus chakra, sits above the navel and below the rib cage. The Sanskrit name for this chakra is *manipura,* and its associated color is yellow. This chakra governs trust in self and honoring your own instincts. When you feel something in your gut, it is the solar plexus chakra activating. The element associated with the solar plexus chakra is fire, its associated sound is *ram*, and its lotus has ten petals.

The fourth chakra, known as the heart chakra, is located at the heart. The Sanskrit name for this chakra is *anahata*. The color associated with this area is green, the color associated with healing. The heart chakra correlates directly to the cardiac plexus, and it governs your ability to love and be loved. The element associated with this chakra is ether. The sound associated with it is *yam*, and its lotus has twelve petals.

The first four chakras of the body are considered to govern the earth self, which is why they have physical elements governing each chakra. The remaining three chakras enter the spiritual space and therefore are not governed by elements. Once the first four chakras are opened (meaning their associated petals have opened), we can experience the joy of the following chakras.

The fifth chakra, called the throat chakra, is located at the throat and corresponds to the laryngeal plexus and thyroid. Its associated color is blue. The throat chakra governs your ability to be heard as well as to speak your truth. When we do not speak honestly or from a loving manner, our throat chakra becomes blocked, resulting in sore throats or other throat issues. The Sanskrit name for this chakra is *vishuddha*. It is associated with the sound *hum*, and its lotus has sixteen petals.

The sixth chakra, called the third eye chakra, is located between and slightly above the eyebrows. This chakra corresponds directly to the cavernous plexus and the pineal gland. The Sanskrit name for this chakra is *ajna*, and its lotus has two petals. The associated color is indigo, and its sound is *om*. This is the place where we are more able to see into the spiritual realm and is often referred to as our spiritual center.

The seventh chakra, known as the crown chakra, is actually located at the very top of the head and slightly above it. Some consider it our connection to the heavens, as it is the last place to close when we come to earth, leaving behind what we know as the soft spot of a baby's head. The Sanskrit name for this chakra is *sahasrara*. Its color is violet or white, and there are no petals in this chakra—when it is open and expanded, it is instead the open fifty-petal lotus above our heads. The sound associated with this chakra is either *om* or silence.

When each chakra is fully opened and the petals bloom, the person experiences something known as *kundalini shakti*, a primal energy that begins at the base of the spine and moves upward through the body/*shushumna* (the energetic spine). This is an awakening of the primal energy through the body generally occurring through practices such as yoga, meditation, tantra, or yantra.

✽ Practice: Turn the Chakras On and Up

Many describe the chakras as wheels spinning in each particular area. The color associated with an energy center radiates throughout the spinning wheel. To clean and clear the energy in each chakra, imagine a circle spinning in each space as we go through them. When you think of the color, however, imagine the color coming through the way a stoplight illuminates as it changes from green to yellow to red. The light doesn't fade; it shines strong and bright through the bulb until the next light shines. There is a chakra cleaning meditation on my website you can get to for free (click on the CDs link at emilyafrancisbooks.com and play the chakra meditation). In that particular meditation, I go through each space with different shapes and subtleties. In the exercise here, I don't want you to think subtle colors—I want you to light up brightly.

Begin sitting upright with your spine straight. You can sit in a chair or cross-legged on the floor. Place the palms facing up in your lap or over your knees. Gently tuck your chin in but not down, allowing the top of the spine through the neck to open. Place the tip of your tongue on the roof of the mouth with the tip of the tongue starting just behind the two front teeth. Now pull the tongue back until you feel a mountain and ridge at the roof of the mouth. Place the tip in the middle of that mountain in the front area of the roof of your mouth at the point where the ridge begins. This activates the energy channel that runs down the front of the face, the front of the body, and through the spine.

Bring your intention to the very base of the spine at the tailbone. Now allow whatever size spinning wheel that fits your body to show itself to you. Turn the wheel in a direction that feels natural. From behind the spinning wheel, turn on your red light. How brightly does your red light shine? Do you see any spots or darkness in this area? This is the root chakra, your root into the earth space. This area is attached to finances and other earthly materials. Keep your red light on and now bring your awareness into the soul area, just at the triangle shaped bone (the sacrum) that sits in your low back. Imagine your spinning wheel in this area. See the color orange turn on and shine through this spinning wheel. This governs the area that not only houses the reproductive organs but the space of creativity as well. When you produce something otherworldly and have no idea how you came up with something so grand, it's because this area is open and in communication with the spirit realm. Let that orange light shine bright from your back to the front side. Allow the wheel to continue spinning; the red and orange colors both shine through their wheels. Next bring your awareness into the solar plexus above your navel and below the ribs. Turn the yellow light on and allow it to shine bright through this space. This is all about your ability to trust your own instinct. Trusting your gut lives right here. What color yellow is shining through this space? How is the wheel spinning? How big is your wheel? How open and connected are you to your own intuition? If you do not yet trust your instincts, ask that the yellow light shine so bright that it obliterates any self-doubt. This space must become open and free from doubt in order for you to truly get to the place where you are able to receive the guidance from the spirit realm. When I say "Collect your data and then trust your gut," it is exactly from this solar plexus chakra that will allow this to happen.

Move your awareness up into the center of your chest, to your heart chakra. This is about being able to give and receive love. Allow the color green to shine its light behind the heart space from the back of your body. Shine it all the way through to the front of your physical body. This is the space where you leave the earthly feelings and transcend into a higher consciousness of operation. It feels nothing like the strong energy of the solar plexus; it is softer, kinder, and timid at times and powerful at others. It is presence, and it changes with your every thought and feeling. This is the space where love lives. Green represents the color for healing. Allow your green light to shine so bright that it outshines any doubt or sorrow. Allow your heart space to free up and feel the healing and loving energy spinning in this space with a comfort that is not too overwhelming. Next up, the blue light turns on at the throat. This is the throat chakra. This is the area where we learn to speak up, speak our truth, and stand up for ourself and others. This is the area where we can learn to trust our own wisdom and share it kindly. Feel the blue light shine through from the back of the neck into the throat, clearing away any debris that may have settled into this space during the times in your life when you lacked the courage to speak up. This is the space of personal power and ownership. Taking responsibility for your thoughts and actions and setting clear intentions and boundaries emanate from this chakra. Be clear in this space and allow your spinning wheel to gently purify the thyroid and the parathyroid glands. Gently move into the third eye and turn on the indigo light. This is the space in which we open to the spirit realm in communication, connection, and sight beyond the physical. Allow the indigo to penetrate the area just above and between the eyebrows. If it is overwhelming, ask that the third eye open at a pace that feels right to you. Finally, open up the crown of your head. Shine the violet light from a few inches below the soft spot on your own head and up and out straight into the sky. Open to Spirit in this space and trust that you are exactly where you are meant to be in this time and space. Let the light shine up and out of you.

Now start again with the root chakra. Shine only one light at a time. Shine the red light and then turn it off, now shine the orange light and off, the yellow light on and off, the green light, the blue light, the indigo light and the violet light. Go through the lighting of the chakras again beginning at the base and working your way up. Now turn them higher in their vibration: When you move up the chakras, imagine them spinning both directions at the same time and keep them on as you move up through the seven chakras. Imagine the spinning wheels turning to the right and left at the same time, multidimensional and lit brightly from behind. Feel yourself activate at a whole new elevated level of being. As each light turns on, this time let them continue shining. The red turns on and shines through you. It stays on as the orange light shines through you and also stays on. The yellow light shines bright and remains shining. Into the heart/green, throat/blue, third eye/indigo, and crown/violet. All of your spinning wheels are spinning both directions, and every light is on and shining through. Keep them as you add more light. Start from your feet. Feel a vibrant white light snake its way from the soles of your feet up your body. Through each color. Traveling up and around through the spine as it slithers up through every color, taking the color into it as it absorbs itself into the great white light. It continues up all the way through your entire body and out through the crown. The white light brightens every single part of your body. You are now bathed in a billowing sensation of soft white light. The colors that are on gently swirl together and join with the white until it all turns simple white. Stay in this white light of peace and purity for as long as you want. When you are ready, turn the white down slightly but not off. Keep it with you as you continue with your day. Operate from that space of purity and kindness. Give thanks and visit this meditation often. This is a beautiful and powerful way to level up with your energy.

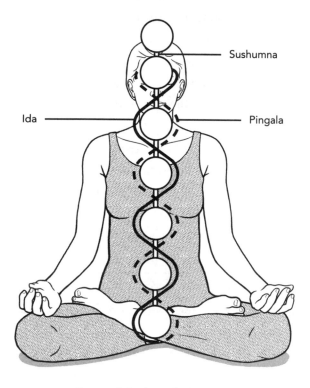

Figure 6: Body with the Nadis

The Nadis

In India, the energy pathways known as nadis (different from the Chinese meridians) are believed to be all over the entire body, numbering something like 72,000 total. In both Chinese and Ayurvedic systems, disease is considered to be the result of a blocked pathway in the body's energetic flow. The nadis are associated physically with the lymphatic, digestive, circulatory, and respiratory systems and house the energy of the physical, subtle, and causal (factors connected to illness) bodies. The nadis connect at various points of higher intensity known as the *nadichakras*. The three basic nadis through which all of the nadis originate are:

1. Ida (left)—This channel begins to the left of the muladhara chakra or root chakra. It passes up through the chakras to the third eye ajna chakra. It flows in curves as opposed to straight lines from one chakra to the next. This channel purifies the mind and body. It is the energy of mental processes including the left nostril and the right side of the brain. It is considered the feminine side.
2. Pingala (right)—This channel also begins at the root chakra and ends at the third eye but begins on the right side. It opens the right nostril and left side of the brain. This is the masculine side of the body. This nadi represents vitality and strength.
3. Sushumna (center)—This is the energetic spine. Think of it as an energetic tube that runs through the body's center line. It is within the sushumna that the seven main chakras are housed, and it is the location in which kundalini shakti can be awakened. Blocks in these nadis can present as physical illness and result in a disconnect within the ability to feel, empathize, and connect deeply with others.

⌘ Practice: Alternate Nostril Breathing

The best option for balancing these three areas is a practice known as alternate nostril breathing. At all times we have one dominant nostril that is more open than the other. In a healthy person, the dominant nostril changes every three hours. Alternate nostril breathing is ideal to encourage openness and balance of the brain through the nostrils. It helps free any blocked energy and balance out the ida, pingala, and the sushumna.

Do this practice with your right hand. The left hand can rest on the lap, palm facing up. If you want to connect the left thumb and first finger, you can make a beneficial mudra (hand position). With the right hand tuck the index and middle finger into the palm and use your right thumb for the right nostril and the right ring and pinky fingers to close the left nostril. The inhale and the hold are for a count of four. The exhales are double that amount to a count of eight. Begin and end with the left side of the nostril.

Exhale through both nostrils to begin.

With the right thumb, close the right nostril, and inhale through the left nostril for a count of four. Close both nostrils and hold the breath (right thumb over right nostril, left ring finger and pinky over the left nostril) for a count of four.

Exhale through the right nostril for a count of eight.

Inhale through the right nostril for a count of four.

Close both sides and hold the breath for a count of four.

Exhale through the left nostril for a count of eight.

That completes one full round. Try to repeat this at least four times through. Once you do the final exhale through the left nostril, bring the hands down and breathe slowly and deeply through both nostrils. Notice the feeling of your mind, and the openness of the nostrils. Note that in the yoga-style practice, we inhale four, hold the breath for sixteen, and exhale eight. For the purposes of this book, inhale four, hold four, and exhale eight.

Yoga

Yoga is a physical, spiritual, and emotional practice founded in India and is a significant part of Ayurveda as a whole. It helps strengthen the body and mind and balances all the body's energy systems. Yoga, yoke, or union is a practice that unites the physical self, the conscious self, and the higher self through practice. Yoga honors all religions but claims none. There is so much more to yoga than simply doing poses; those asanas, or physical movements, are only one aspect of yoga as a practice in daily life. There are four main branches.

Bhakti yoga: This is a devotional practice of yoga with love as the center of all actions and thoughts. The goal is to purify the heart. This is considered the easiest and safest of the four paths. In this practice, when emotions come up, the aim is to simply learn to channel the energy into something devotional rather than attempt to change the feeling into something else or push it away. The foundation of this practice is prayer, chanting, japa meditation (repeating God's name), ceremony, and ritual. Followers of this system believe there are four cases in which a person would turn to bhakti as practice: (1) when everything in their life has failed and they turn to God as refuge

(2) curiosity (3) seeking gain in spiritual devotion, knowledge, or wealth as they believe God to hear all petitions of favors are approached with love and devotion, and (4) the desire to love and serve God without attachment to the self or the material world.

Karma yoga: In karma yoga, the aim is to engage in selfless service that results in clearing one's karma. This is the yoga of action, and the goal is to purify the ego. It can be practiced anywhere at any and all times when you choose to act with the intention of offering to God. It is renouncing personal desires and acting in a way that is unselfish. There are three types of karma: *sanchita,* the actions from your past in this life and the previous lives, which may be unresolved actions or consequences that you are accountable for; *parabda,* action in the present tense, or what you are currently doing in this life and the results of this present action; and *agami* karma, which is about future actions that are a result of the present actions you are engaging in currently. As we attempt to clear karma from the past, we unavoidably create more of it. The goal is learning to behave in a way that does not incur more karma through your behaviors and choices and in learning to take control of your behaviors. To do this requires becoming fully present and aware of everything you choose with the understanding that there is a consequence attached to every action.

Jnana yoga: This is considered the most direct of all the four paths. Its goal is the gaining of knowledge and the purification of the intellect. This is the most difficult path as it uses the intellect to reach enlightenment. It requires constant self-analysis and deep inquiry. A person must be grounded and highly studied in the other disciplines before attempting this specific avenue of study.

Raja yoga: Also called ashtanga yoga, this is a practice of mind control. The goal is to purify the astral body and learn to control the mind. Certain techniques are used to bring the mind under your control to get to higher states of consciousness. There are eight limbs of raja yoga. This is where the yoga practices we understand and associate with the idea of yoga in the West are housed. This covers physical movements (asanas), breathing (pranayama), meditation, and so on. Kundalini and hatha yoga are subdivisions of raja yoga.

Meditation

Meditation is a state of consciousness in which thoughts are able to flow without attachment or judgment. Because I discuss meditation and offer practices throughout this text, I will simply list the health benefits of having a meditation practice and then offer a very simple meditation burst, as I call them. When a person regularly engages in a meditation practice, they can experience an increase in relaxation and reduction in stress. They also learn how to handle stress more efficiently. Emotional health becomes a more active part of life. Through meditation, we learn how to navigate life's challenges without so much attachment to the issues that arise. We become more self-aware of the world around us and how we fit into it. Having a meditation practice helps us act with more kindness toward ourselves and others. When we begin to treat ourselves with more respect, we begin to treat the outside world much the same way. We become more consciously aware of life. We begin to value our life and the lives of all living things more than we used to. Meditation can help with pain control and improve the quality of sleep at night and rest times during the day. It helps us to slow down and chill out even outside of our practice.

Taking time out to help connect to your higher self is paramount for increasing health and vitality. It helps put things into perspective. You do not need to meditate for an hour; it is beneficial even in small doses. You can keep the time short, but do your best to keep it up daily.

✻ PRACTICE: MEDITATION BURSTS

These little gems only last about thirty seconds to a minute. You don't have to take your shoes off or sit in any particular place or position. Just take one step back from whatever is in front of you and close your eyes. Exhale fully and completely. Inhale one single word that represents what you want to bring in, something positive you need right now. Exhale and release one word that represents what you'd like to release right now. Repeat the same words that you've chosen in and out for three to ten repetitions. Open your eyes and see when you take that step back in if you don't feel just a little more centered and ready to reengage. For those who use a tapping practice, pairing this meditation with that technique to the collar bone or sternum can amplify this practice tenfold.

An Example A Day For A Week:

Inhale love ... exhale fear.

Inhale peace ... exhale frustration.

Inhale gentleness ... exhale violence.

Inhale health ... exhale negativity.

Inhale kindness ... exhale sadness.

Inhale calm ... exhale worry.

Inhale creativity ... exhale blocks.

Visualization

Visualization is a form of meditation and psychotherapy as its own practice. When we visualize with a specific intention for improving mental clarity, focus, concentration, or specific movements (such as a sport), the desired outcome begins its manifestation in our minds. Once we set the tone for what we want the scenario to look like, we play it in our minds like a movie and then set it on repeat for the best effects. Visualization is a specific practice that can enhance an outcome.

⌘ Practice: Visualization for Peace and Release

Lie down someplace comfortable. Close your eyes and soften your face. Breathe out slowly and deeply, and then take a long inhale that fills the lungs. Exhale and send a wave of relaxing energy down your body and out through your feet. Set the breaths to be long, silent, and relaxing. Close your eyes. Now go deeply into your mind and imagine yourself in a meadow. Feel the soft green grass between your toes as you walk toward a small stream. By the stream is a large, thick tree. Imagine yourself lying down with your head near the base of the tree right next to the stream. Lie down here, and in your mind's eye, begin to explore your surroundings without moving your head or your body. Take in the smell of the fresh air, the sounds from birds chirping up above and from the stream. Gently drop one arm down and allow the hand to reach into the water, allowing the gentle flow to run between your fingers. Notice that one single leaf detaches from the tree above and begins to float gently side to side as it slowly makes its way down. It lands in the water just above your fingertips. Open your palm up to catch that leaf and hold it in the palm of your hand. In your mind's eye, notice every little vein and line on that leaf. From far away it looks like a nondescript green leaf, but upon closer inspection you see that it is gloriously detailed. Keeping your body still and your eyes closed, I invite you now to take one item from your life that weighs heavily on you. Place that one thing directly on that leaf. Hold it in your hand for a moment as the energy of that one item attaches itself to the leaf and separates itself from you. Now open your hand up and allow that leaf to float away. As you release that leaf and that stressor, take a deep breath in and out. Savor how you feel in this exact moment without that attachment. Keeping your eyes closed, do an internal body scan and notice how your whole body feels without that item in your life. Now slowly begin to bring your awareness back to the air around you and feel the air on your skin as you start to notice the surrounding smells and sounds. Gently wiggle your fingers and your toes as you prepare to open your eyes and come back into your daily life. Move slowly and with intention not to bring that item back with you. You've let it go. I want you to keep this new lightness and wonder in your body and mind. Gently open your eyes and return.

Affirmations

An affirmations is similar to a visualization except it isn't a visual product but a verbal practice that sets the mind to a new tone and intention regarding any specific subject matter. Affirmations can be extremely powerful in changing the patterns set in our mind. What we may not realize is that the power of this practice does not discriminate between positive and negative intentions. Remember, there is always a choice. Be careful about negative affirmations. For example, I was at the airport catching a morning flight. I decided to run to the rest room before they called my row to board. While washing my hands, I looked up to see a TSA agent come to a nearby sink to wash her hands. I didn't think anything of it until I heard her say very affirmatively "I look so fat" under her breath. Then she let out the saddest sigh, as if to lock into her body the shameful beatdown she administered upon herself. I looked over at her and saw her making sad faces at herself in the mirror. What she didn't realize was that she was actually practicing the art of affirmation but in the most damaging way: she was affirming to herself that she *is* fat and "should" be ashamed. Through her practice, she was literally locking into each cell of her body that she was not enough. The magnitude of damage she was doing to herself was totally lost on her until I stood in her way and interrupted her dialogue. I looked her in the eye and said, "You look fantastic." She was embarrassed that I heard her and that I had the gumption to speak up. I continued, "Do you realize that if anything should happen to you, you would wish to God you looked exactly like you do right now?" Her face was full of surprise at that quick *Aha!* moment. Not breaking eye contact, I said, "You are beautiful. You are strong. You are powerful. And it's time to change that dialogue." Her eyes teared up and she acknowledged that yes, it was time. I left almost in tears myself. It was painful in my own body to bear witness to such damaging and self-harming behavior. She wasn't just berating herself; she was looking at herself in the mirror and giving a direct affirmation. It was damaging to her whole being, and she had no idea the magnitude of power this tone sets off inside herself.

Affirmations are powerful. It is entirely our choice whether we make them healing or damaging. We have got to take our power back and use our inner voice for something good.

"Every cell in my body is reprogramming itself now to function at healthy, optimum levels."

Remember: You are smart. You are beautiful. You are powerful. It is time to take back your power. It is time to change that dialogue. Repeat after me: "Every cell in my body is reprogramming itself to function at healthy, optimum levels." This is an Emily Francis original, and it has served me very well through the years. Now I happily pass it on to you.

Chapter 10
Hands-On Healing Practices

The following section introduces hands-on healing practices including Reiki, Therapeutic Touch, Healing Touch, Seven Rays, and Deeksha. Before offering these practices, it is important to understand the intention behind hands-on energy healing.

One key question to ask is "Who is the healer?" Let me answer: It is Spirit/God/Goddess/the Universe—whatever name you choose. It was not and is not me who is doing the healing. That being said, when it comes to your own body being able to heal from within, *you* are the healer. You and Spirit are the healers. "I am the healer of my life," "I am the healer of my body," and "I choose to heal," are true and powerful statements I encourage you to use as daily mantras that carry immense sacred energy to perpetuate your greatest health. However, keep in mind that referring to yourself as a healer to anyone else robs the person(s) you are working with of their own experience of empowerment through their own healing. When you proclaim it is *you* who heals, you take away someone's power and claim it as your own. Remember that it is each person's own body/mind/energy/spirit/soul connection within every cell and fiber of their being that allows healing to occur—no one else can do that. When it comes to any sort of bodywork or healing practice, I open myself up to Spirit, who works through and with me. I give the glory to God and my Spirit team. I like to call them a "team" because there are many. I am grateful they choose me to work through, and I get the feeling that if I took advantage of the beautiful relationship between us, they would choose someone else—someone humbler—to work with instead. My job is to be the vessel, not receive top billing.

That said, many gifted people refer to themselves as healers, which is perfectly fine as it is their choice. I may engage in healing practices, and I may refer to someone else as a healer. Those are different statements from a proclamation that I am the *source* for someone's healing. Normally when I hear someone refer to themselves as a healer, it simply indicates to me that they may be fairly new to healing work and haven't settled on a better way to describe the practices they engage in. I see it in quite a few bios, e.g., the first line is "I am a healer." Again, calling oneself a healer is a personal choice and not necessarily a reflection on anyone's work. When we know better, we do better; when we understand deeper, we present our gifts differently. When I find people such as Dr. Upledger (creator of Upledger Craniosacral Therapy), whose very first rule to all students is that you are never the healer, I instantly feel as if I have found a kindred spirit.

The way someone presents themselves and their work is very telling. Pay attention to more than just the wording someone chooses. Other things to note are how much money they expect you to spend and how many times they suggest you visit. There are some incredibly gifted healing practitioners out there who are generally humble and very loving in their energy who also set clear boundaries. You may feel very drawn to these people and hopefully feel safe in their space. There should be no expectation that they give their work at a discounted rate or for free. These people know they do great work and are firm in what they expect to receive in exchange. They take their work seriously and consider it a sacred practice. Therefore, they do not overcharge or undercharge. They usually are aware of the going rate for that particular practice and will usually stay close to the average. As well, they will not insist on you returning more than is truly necessary to help you shift and heal. Often times they will even refer you to someone else they believe can help you further. These gifted healers are not selfish; they truly have your healing interests above their own financial agendas. They are not constantly pushing a different service they provide.

Sadly, there are also a lot of people whose primary goal is making money. Those people often tell you to come back several times for a variety of reasons or treatments. They might even exaggerate their level of training or work outside of their scope of practice. I consider people like this to be my nemesis and there are plenty of them. Of all the advice offered throughout this book, the most important is to always check a person's credentials. While this isn't possible when consulting a psychic, medium, or person who does channeling, in energy practices such as massage, craniosacral therapy, and other bodywork specialties, it is the most important thing you can do. If the person is trained, there should be no issue in showing you certifications and a state or national license, if applicable. If I've learned anything in my child's healing process, it is that you *must* be bold enough to ask to see credentials and know whether a practitioner has sufficient training as well. People do not offer the truth willingly if they are not properly trained, and some will take advantage of your trust and lack of familiarity.

Reiki

Reiki is a form of hands-on healing that uses universal life force energy. It is similar to the laying-on of hands mentioned in the Bible. Reiki's creator, Mikao Usui, is from Japan, where it is frequently used in the hospitals. There are currently several US government grants backing the research and application of Reiki practice in complementary medicine. Reiki is from the highest level of spiritual awareness. A person opens up their body to be a vessel for the Universe's healing energy to the person receiving it. When practicing, the Reiki practitioner may offer a prayer, surround the space with light, set the intention, and offer themselves as a clear and open channel for unconditional love and Reiki energy. The recipient can feel a number of things when receiving. They can see colors, images, or feel an unexplainable calm. Massive amounts of healing can occur during Reiki sessions. Because Reiki is the way in which I am trained to work with someone's energy body, I can give the most accurate firsthand information regarding this practice.

Therapeutic Touch (TT)

Therapeutic Touch was created by Dolores Kreiger, PhD, RN, and is an energy work practice that uses a more clinical approach. While nurses are most often associated with this work, anyone can train in this particular practice. Currently, more clinical research is being done to back the results of this practice because its practitioners are mainly health-care professionals. TT offers treatment of several medical conditions by using the hands to manipulate the human energy field above a patient's skin. Many times (if not all the time), a practitioner does not directly touch skin but instead holds their hands above the recipient to work.

Healing Touch

Created by Janet Mentgen, RN, Healing Touch is a heart-centered hands-on energy practice that helps balance the human energy system for health in all areas—emotional, physical, spiritual, and mental. In this practice, hands are placed directly on a recipient's skin to help clear and heal through their energy system.

Key Differences between the Three Hands-On Energy Practices

Some differences between the three practices of Reiki, Healing Touch, and Therapeutic Touch are that Reiki is passed through an attunement from a teacher who was attuned through the lineage of either Mikao Usui or Mrs. Takata. Healing Touch and Therapeutic Touch do not require any attunement but do require proper training and a specific set of hours of practice, as both were created by nurses. Reiki allows the flow of energy, whereas Therapeutic Touch and Healing Touch direct the flow of energy. All three hands-on healing approaches can be applied to a recipient of any religious tradition.

Sacred Fatigue

Engaging in any hands-on energy practices can be really powerful but also taxing. Someone once said to me that whenever we practice Reiki, we also receive it at the same time. Therefore, we don't get tired when engaging in the practice. From personal experience, I have to say that while I may not get tired while I'm in the healing space, I get very fatigued after it's done, though it's a sacred fatigue, not simply exhaustion. In fact, *sacred fatigue* is a perfect description for the work I engage in. At one point in my practice, I had to step back from energy work because so much transfer was happening to my body as a result. I worked on a friend's friend who just had surgery on her liver for cancer. I put my hands over that space, and when I got home later that day it looked like I had been cut across my own liver; that scar remained for several weeks. I decided at that time to take a break and stop my hands-on work; I was unintentionally taking way too much onto myself. It is easy to assume that I must not have been doing things correctly if I was transferring like that, but it's important to remember that there are no set rules with energy work, even when we try to implement them. The way one person can transfer or open up for energy will likely be totally different from the next because practice is extremely individual to each person.

Energy work can be exhausting, just as it can be liberating and freeing. It can be incredibly healing to both the recipient and the conduit. It does not mean when you are feeling high and healed that you did it correctly nor when you feel like you traveled down into the recipient's pain with them that you were doing something wrong. It's the nature of the beast. You are in their energy space and you are also in the energy space of the whole cosmic consciousness. When you are that open, you don't necessarily get a map that shows you how to avoid transfer. No matter which sensations I feel the most following a session, there is still a certain holy fatigue in coming together with Spirit for the greater good of someone else. While many would welcome that kind of work space, it is not something I could do all day long, every day. For me, the energy can be too much when held for too long of a time. I am an intense person as it is (I'm a Scorpio with an 11/11 birthday—seriously intense), sitting for long periods and working from that high of a space with different bodies isn't the right thing for me to achieve a good sense of balance. I know this about myself and set my work accordingly.

When putting hands on someone with the intention to allow energy to pass through you, there are some fundamental rules. You must create a sacred space and set your intentions on what is and is not allowed in your healing space and practice. You are the hands, and you are the open and clear vessel through which Spirit can work. Be open, be clear, and do what you need to close the line of energy when you are done. Be sure to have an opening sequence that you follow as well as a closing sequence to end. Be clear in your intentions. You are in charge of this space. Try not to take on the other person's energy, but also don't pretend that it's impossible. Regardless of how energy moves, it is always along the path of least resistance. Finish with a clearing of the energy and a stopping of the channel. I do a big Z with my hand down to the ground and bang my palm against the floor to signal the energy is done. Then I give thanks for each time that Spirit allows me to be their hands. When I leave the space and wash my hands, I wash for a good long time, giving my hands and forearms a good scrubbing. I simultaneously give thanks for allowing me to work with the spirits and ask that the energy now remove from me and bring me back down into my earthly body and awareness.

Deeksha

Though I have only received the Deeksha blessing twice, it was lovely each time. Created by Sri Bhagavan, it is considered a blessing of oneness and from my understanding, it is also used to clear your karma from past lives. When I received the blessing, it was extremely calm and welcomed. I sat on the floor under a blanket and listened to beautiful music while waiting for the Deeksha giver to place his hands over my head. Deeksha itself does not have any religious affiliation; it is simply a blessing of oneness. Typically, it is given through the hands onto the recipient's crown to facilitate awakening. When I received it, it left a sense of peace for a very long time afterwards. I personally believe that it did clear energy from the past.

As I did research on this topic, however, I had to look at both sides of the findings. I was able to find reactions and experiences of Deeksha that were quite different from my own. Some people reported experiencing psychosis after receiving the blessing. Some felt very ill and developed pain in their bodies. As I understand it, this blessing is intended to help clear karma from this life and past lives. That might be a very heavy load to carry. Try to approach such a blessing with respect and preparation. Find a solid practitioner who knows what they are doing. Do the necessary preparations to be as clean in your own body and mind before the blessing is given. Eat clean, meditate, and set your intentions for what you are hoping to clear and to gain through this blessing. Talk with the practitioner before you do this. Be sure you are on the same page and that you are clear with your intention to heal.

Seven Rays

The Seven Rays of this healing correspond to seven Ascended Masters. An Ascended Master was once human and is now a high-level spiritual being on the other side. Our greatest example of an Ascended Master is Christ himself. In Seven Rays healing, we use a certain protocol to call in each of the different rays according to their role in bringing energy from the heavens to the recipient. One hand receives the energy while the other hand directs the energy ray into the person receiving. I have had incredibly profound results from this technique. A man who was addicted to drugs once came to me for what turned out to be an extremely intense session. He was shaking, sweating, screaming, and crying; it was like the darkness was being removed from him. I even resorted to using holy water and using sea salt to absorb some of the negative energy that was being thrown off from his body. One particular ray of the seven took the addiction and darkness and blew it out of his body. It was extremely intense for both of us, but the rewards far outweighed the effort. He left the session and stayed sober for quite some time after.

Pranic Healing

Pranic Healing is a style of energy healing originating from the Philippines. It is a no-touch energy practice that works with the body's internal prana for healing, through which the body's ability to heal itself is used through breath, energy, and intention. It is widely used around the world and is a powerful healing practice.

Scalar Energy

Because we have not had the terminology or basic foundations of the concept of chi/ki/prana, the West is behind in understanding the magnitude of this powerful, life force energy. In order for the Western mindset to be more receiving of such a concept, it has been put into different labeling. The clinical term behind this energy is now presented as scalar energy. Taking that many steps further, I had the pleasure of interviewing Tom Paladino on my radio show, scalar energy researcher and creator of scalar light technology. He and other brilliant researchers and partners developed instruments that are able to capture and control the scalar energy in order to destroy pathogens within the body. This means that the technology they have developed (and research to back up findings will be included in the resource section of this book) can effectively disassemble and destroy bacteria, viruses, and fungi. Scalar energy is not electricity. In fact, the energy that they have been able to capture on film and work with is longitudinal, seen as a double helix. The instruments he developed are able to capture and control the double helix (that's what a scalar wave is) in order to destroy various pathogens. These instruments have destroyed pathogens such as the herpes virus and Lyme bacteria. They have research at a clinic in Delhi, India working with more than two-thousand HIV patients in destroying the virus. Visit www.scalarlight.com for more research and results into this practice. This is something that requires an open mind and a willingness to receive healing that comes from a form that might be difficult to understand. I encourage you to be open to the possibilities that are available to you and those that you love who have not been able to successfully treat various conditions.

The Aura

While the meridian channels and the nadis run throughout the inside of the body, the aura is the energy we carry from our physical body outward and the frequency of energy that surrounds us. Generally, the aura is egg-shaped and extends about three feet out from our bodies. There are people who can see all kinds of things within someone's energy aura. Some people claim to see shapes and densities where it is healthiest or has been compromised. Some people are able to see colors that surround the body.

How you are able to perceive and interpret someone's energy whether through sight, sound, feeling, or instinct will determine how you can relate to a person's external energy. Once you begin to work within your strongest abilities, understanding the outside energy body becomes a little bit easier to identify with. If you do have the gift of vision, you may well be able to see the colors that emanate from a person. There is special photography that can capture the colors and light of the aura. If you are more likely to sense someone's energy, you will likely be able to gauge how you feel in their presence more than you can see what is vibrating around them. We will discuss the four Clairs in the spirit section. Once you know which gift is your best gift, that is how you can begin to work with understanding someone's energy or your own energy through the lens that is best fit for you.

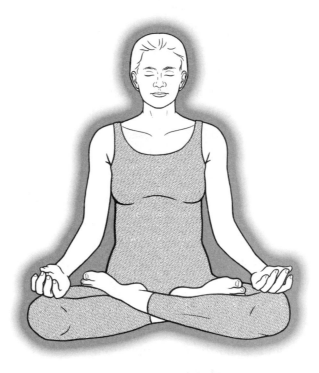

Figure 7: Aura

⌘ Practice: Feel Your Aura

Sit crossed-legged either on a blanket or cushion to make your hips comfortable. Your buttocks should be on the edge of the blanket or cushion and your feet and legs on the floor. Be sure your spine is straight and that the chin is slightly tucked under but not down. Place your hands either together as if in prayer at the chest or with the palms facing up on your knees. Close your eyes and begin to slow down the breathing. Envision four lines of energy from your body. The first wall or line of energy comes from the front center line of your entire body. The second line of energy comes from the center line out from the spine. The other two energy lines come from your sides. Four perfect lines all emanate from your body, from the skin outward to the imagined lines outside yourself. Inhale and feel the energy expand however far it can. Exhale and feel the lines come back into your body. With each breath, allow the energy to expand more and more but don't strain—only go to the place where you can feel it in your body and imagine it in your mind. This energy space is in your field of energy. This is where your aura expands in this moment. Depending on how long you stay with this process, notice any colors, shapes, symbols, webbing, or anything within the space as you breathe and expand and release. Stay in this space until you feel comfortable with the images you received. When ready, simply come back into your physical body, feel the air on your skin, feel the floor beneath you, and slowly open your eyes.

Energy Transfer

In massage school, we did a practice to understand the energy that can transfer through touch. One person sat in the middle of a circle. The rest of the class sat around that person in the center. One person went out into the hall and drew a piece of paper that listed an emotion to feel. The objective was to come from behind the person sitting down (who had their eyes closed) and put your hands on the tops of their shoulders, thinking of the emotion while trying to send it into the person. Almost every single person guessed the correct emotion just through touch and being able to perceive thoughts and intention. When you open yourself up to touch and to feeling someone's energy, you can almost instinctually feel what they are thinking. Remember, the emotional body and energy body are not the same things but are very closely woven. They always overlap in the energetic space.

It is important to be able to understand and differentiate the energy space from the emotional space. Learning to discern the way something feels to you without contact is an energy component that can be of great benefit once you learn how to use it as your superpower instead of your kryptonite. You can practice the way we did in massage school by touching someone and sending a particular feeling to them. Do this as an interactive practice, however, and don't do it without consulting the other person, getting consent, and setting clear boundaries.

Chapter 11

Energy Cords, the Empath, and Psychic Protection

E nergy cords are connections between us and people who have been in our lives whom we share a connection with. Generally speaking, energy cords can be perfectly healthy to have between friends and lovers. It's when a person in your life has caused you pain, or is toxic, that will require intervention to eliminate the connection between you.

Energy Cords

Have you randomly thought of someone or even dreamt of someone you haven't spoken to in a long time, and they called you out of the blue right after or during your thought? Or say you've gone through a breakup with someone that leaves you heartbroken and devastated for weeks to months, but one day you finally realize you don't miss them anymore and you like someone else … and that's exactly when that person comes calling and decides they want you back. What both scenarios have in common are energy cords between you and the other person: on a very subtle level, you decided to pull your cord, and they felt that pull. In reality, there is no "out of the blue"—what you're feeling is the energy frequency that goes from one person to another.

Whenever we connect on a deeper level with someone in friendship, partnership, and so on, we create a cord that binds us to each other in some aspect. If the other person is an intimate partner, the cord is much stronger. For this reason, we need to think before becoming intimate with someone whom we are not terribly invested in. When we connect with someone on an intimate physical level, a cord is created and connected whether you acknowledge it or not. This is partially why I believe that even if we pretend that we don't care what happens after we are intimate with someone, it's never really that simple. We connected ourselves to the other person through that experience. And what's neat about the energy connection is that when you find yourself thinking of someone, it is likely because they were thinking about you. Energy cords run both ways. It's a level of frequency that is so subtle despite its activity that it's hard to fully appreciate how powerful it can be.

Cord Cutting

This practice has many interpretations. Some people think of cord cutting in the energetic realm, and others consider it as something that takes place in the interpersonal realm between yourself and someone who doesn't bring anything positive to your life. Some people want to cut the cord between themselves and negative energy itself, not necessarily from any one person but a heavy and one-sided attachment from the spirit realm (referred to as cutting energy cords or cutting etheric cords). It's also possible to cut cords between you and certain painful memories. Just as we cut the cord between mother and child after birth, so too can we cut cords to things born out of fear, trauma, spite, or anything that does not serve us. Cords can be formed from a space in the subconscious and can be a result of a manipulation or need for control over something or someone. There are spells and prayers to help you cut the cords that bind you to something.

To help cut cords between myself and a person or situation, I always find it helpful to write on a piece of paper and ask Spirit to help. I then burn the paper to help deliver the messages and send it out into the Universe. I personally add black salt for protection, frankincense to purify, amber to dissolve negative energy, and sage to cleanse and release.

⌘ Practice: Cord Cutting

As you prepare, it is important to get very clear with your intention before you put this practice into motion. Do you truly want to be liberated from this person or situation? Are you ready to walk away without this in your life? Ask yourself honestly and be willing to do your part. Once you engage in this practice, you must be willing to walk away forever. You cannot ask to cut cords and then turn around and change your mind. If you think there's a chance you may one day feel differently, stop here. Only do this practice when you are truly ready to leave something behind and move on with your life.

Be somewhere silent and alone where you will not be interrupted. Sit up with your spine straight, eyes closed, and palms over your heart center or in a prayer position. Imagine the person, feeling, or situation sitting in front of you. They are sitting in the same position you are, almost like a reflection in a mirror, close enough for you to reach out and touch. Notice that from your heart to their heart is a thick rope connecting you two. Say out loud or in your mind your specific intentions for this practice. In your mind's eye, pull out a large pair of scissors and open the scissors to get ready to cut the middle of the cord between the two spaces. Cut the cord that goes from their heart to your heart. Now take the remaining cord that goes from the cut piece into you and pull out the remaining cord that might still be rooted in your heart space. Don't worry about removing anything from them; this is a cord cutting visualization specific to *you*. As well, don't wish harm or anything else on the other person other than the ability to turn their head away peacefully and move beyond this person or situation forever. Don't invest yourself in their happiness, safety, comeuppance, sadness, or anything—only ask to be separated in a way that is healthy and lasting for both involved. After cutting, sit in the space for a bit and notice if you feel any different without that person being attached to you. Reaffirm your choice of disengaging from that person or situation. Trust that what you just did was real and believe it to be true. We don't have to keep everything painful with us; we are in charge of our lives, and the things that bring us pain do not need to be part of it moving forward. You have everything you need to live a happy, healthy, and vibrant existence without being pulled back or down. Your cord is now severed. Walk away freely.

⌘ Practice: Cut, Clear, Disengage, Disconnect

This practice is best done immediately in the moment when either you or someone else says something that attaches to a negative thought or energy. Let's use an easy example: trying to make a break from a toxic person in our lives such that we don't want to hear their name mentioned. Imagine that a friend forgot and brings the toxic person up. Take your fingers through the air and cut in a Z or X shape as you say out loud: "Cut, Clear, Disengage, Disconnect." This immediately cuts the energy and releases the bind. Use this practice as often as necessary.

The Empath

An empath is someone who is highly sensitive to outside energy and can tune in to other people's energy. They can feel emotions, pains, and energy as if it were their own. A lot of information about empath energy and sensitive people is out there on social media these days, but it goes much deeper than a simple explanation that you might be a sensitive person. Being an empath can be the reason some of us get so lost among the collective energies of other people. Being an empath and feeling other people's energy can easily make us feel like we have a first-class ticket on the crazy train, something that is especially true when too many people are around, or someone's energy is particularly chaotic.

Being an empath goes deeper than simply having empathy for someone. The gift of super sensitivity can easily turn from a blessing to a curse when you don't learn how to harness it. Oftentimes empaths become overly sensitive to everything and everyone around them. They can become vulnerable to outside influences and energies, and it can be tough to navigate. They can easily feel things too much, including taking on the pain (physical or emotional) of others, feeling overwhelmed in crowded places, or crying over sad or disturbing news. This kind of feeling can happen whether the sensitive person is told details or not! It can be very intense to carry such a gift/burden.

I remember sitting next to a particularly strong energetic person once at a book talk I attended right after going to a tai chi class. As I sat next to this man, whom I hadn't been introduced to yet, I started experiencing a searing pain in one of my biceps. It became so noticeable that I had to mentally step back and do a quick inventory and body scan of myself to figure out what was going on: "Did I get hurt? Did I pull my bicep? Did something happen that I didn't realize at tai chi?" Once I stepped back mentally, I realized that the pain was not my own. I scanned the room and tapped into the various people to see where it was coming from. I realized it was coming from the guy sitting next to me, so I focused in on his energy and body. When the book talk paused for a break, I asked him if he had any issues with that arm because I was experiencing phantom pains in my own arm, a step I was not particularly comfortable with at the time. Asking him required self-trust and willingness to be vulnerable. He replied, impressed, "Oh yeah, I tore that bicep tendon. It hurts all the time. Can you feel it?" I understood in that moment that although it was fun to be able to feel what someone else was feeling, being an empath in this manner had the potential to weigh heavily on me if I didn't get a handle on it. I couldn't go around taking on people's pains whenever I left the house! But I also wondered how many times I did that anyway without knowing. Too many times the sensitive empaths are unaware that they could easily walk away taking with them someone's pain without even noticing it.

When I was younger and knew nothing about the way of the empath, I tended to follow a cycle of showing up when people needed someone to bear the burden of a sudden trauma that had occurred in their lives. I would stay for as long as they needed me to stay and figuratively swallow their pain and trauma like it was my own situation to handle. I was "all up in it" (a Southern term) with them, in the thick of all the deepest pains they had to deal with. Not once did it occur to me that this was *their* pain, *their* life path, and *their* road to take in order to heal themselves. Instead, I took it on for them; I lightened their load and put myself way out beyond what is necessary to be a good friend. I prided myself on being the one who always showed up when something really bad happened to someone I loved. I even showed up for people I wasn't necessarily close to, as I somehow knew just when to appear and take on their pain. I offered escape routes for their pain, whether it looked like taking them out to get absolutely hammered drunk, sitting and crying with them, or assisting them in whatever needed to be done in their process. I've sat with police detectives and sketch artists to help someone very dear to me create a sketch of the man who did unspeakable things to her as if I were there when it happened. I'm not saying that I should have left each of these people to their own devices when their lives took a hard turn, but I could have avoided taking on the anguish as if it were my own. There is a very fine line between sharing compassion and being compromised.

Back then, I didn't know any better. I thought what I did made me a good friend and that my special gift was to help people cross bridges in their lives. Unfortunately, once those people had gotten to the next level and felt good enough to get up and start living life again, I was still plagued with the pain I had taken on for them. That pain continued to pile on and weigh me down. I began to live my life as a collection of all the really bad stuff that happened around me. Very little of it was ever my own to bear, but I sure was good at taking one for the team. I loaded their weights and burdens onto my own shoulders and traveled the road beside them. I had no idea about boundaries, energetic or otherwise. I didn't know how to clear myself of someone's trauma; nobody teaches this stuff in school!

It took me a very long time to understand what an empath was. It was challenging to learn how to navigate my sensitivities and be there for someone without taking their pain on as my own. In fact, it wasn't really until I began hands-on bodywork that I learned how to harness other people's energy and emotions. Even then, it took many years to be able to refine my skills and use them for the greater good of all involved.

It's unfortunate that the very real issue of pain transferred through energy, intentional or not, is not widely covered or well known. Intentional transfer is of course much stronger, but unintentional transfer probably happens more frequently. It's not the fault of the person who is hurting, of course, so it falls on *you* to know how to handle someone else's energy. I will show you how in the protection area of this chapter.

If you are an empath but haven't learned to work within your special skill set, think of yourself as having a car battery that offers a certain amount of energy. Once that battery runs out, the car won't start, and you'll be stuck on the side of the road by yourself. For the empath, that may mean being knocked out in bed, down for the count. Empaths are beautiful, highly sensitive creatures with a gift of truly understanding someone's pain. Balance it well and it will serve you tremendously. Neglect mindfulness, and that gift will catch you unaware, with ugly results.

✖ PRACTICE: OUTSIDE OF THE BODY SCAN

Earlier we did a practice for ourselves called the body scan, and we learned to do a daily check-in with our bodies to identify any pains or issues. We then went deeper into questioning ourselves about where the pain or issues may be located and their origin. This practice uses the same tuning-in strategy but in exactly the opposite place. With this practice, we learn to do an external scan and tap into energies coming from outside ourselves.

If you find yourself in a space where the energy is running high or overwhelming you, it is important to learn to disconnect yourself from that energy and scan the space to figure out what energy is coming from where. It can be very overwhelming if you are in a space with several people due to how much energy is running wild. Your average person has no concept of how to hold their own energetic space. Stressful people emanate an energy that is difficult for us sensitives to handle.

Begin by doing a scan of whatever space you are in. Gently and momentarily tap into various energies coming from around the space you are in. If you find energy coming from certain people, gently and quickly tap into it so you can trace any lines of heaviness and figure out their source. You can still be there for someone if they need you, but don't take their stuff on and put it into you. Become aware of your own energy lines and hold them in with protection. Don't give away your energy and don't take in their energy. Notice where each heavy space of energy is coming from. Is the person trying to give you their sorrows? Do you feel like you are near an energy vacuum? If so, hold your space and draw your lines. Do not take it in. Be loving and kind, but be firm within your own boundaries of where you end and they begin.

If you are in a room full of people and need to be integrated into this space, the outward scan will be a little different: this time, you are simply collecting energy data. Tap into the collective energy of the room and figure out where you fit into it. Again, you are still protecting the lines of space outlining your energy body and not taking in other people's stuff. Tap into the collective and see what you can offer to it and how best to go about it. While you are in that space, be willing to be totally present to the whole and engage fully. But when it's time to leave the space, be sure you do your own quick body scan and check to be sure you are not taking with you anyone else's energy that they may have unknowingly tried to pour on you.

Protection

I cannot discuss energy without teaching you about the necessary skills to protect yourself. There are many ways in which people choose to open themselves up energetically, and there are just as many ways in which people protect themselves in those highly vulnerable spaces. We don't want to walk away with everyone's pain and sorrows or any negative energy that they might have brought into a space unknowingly. When we open up to the light, there is an equally powerful energetic pull toward the dark that also shows up. We may not even notice it because we have gotten so good at setting the space to be clear of anything like this, but it is always there as an option. Each and every time, it's up to us to choose to work within the light for the greatest good and highest joys of all involved. Clearing the space, setting the intention, and knowing how to protect our space and ourselves is paramount with this work. The best thing to start with is to clear the air by burning sage before anyone enters. It's then a good idea to waft that sage smoke around any person entering the space to set an energetically clean space for working.

Set Your Intention: There are several things you can say while washing your hands before and after working with anyone. This is the time to begin your practice of keeping your energetic space clean and clear. Set the intention to provide the best service you are able to without taking on anyone's energy. Ask whatever higher powers you call upon to help you in assisting your work. Create a protective bubble where you can give energy but are not able to take energy in. You can personally develop any practice, prayer, or intention prior to beginning your work.

Set Your Space: For a space to be protected, you must create it to be that way. There are a number of ways to do this, and there is no single right way. Many people have their own preferred methods of creating sacred and protected spaces. In my own practice, I move my fingers in a circle facing the ceiling as I repeat these words: "I cast a circle around this space that only the highest light may enter." From there, I proceed to use burning sage to clear the space, myself, and anyone who enters.

Sage/Smoke Cleansing: Burning sage is a practice that has been around for an extremely long time. You can use it in the home, in the practice room, on yourself and others. If someone leaves your space and their energy felt funky to you, burn some sage to help escort the energy out of your house. If I have a bundle, I begin by lighting it until I have smoke and then blow out the flame, letting the ashes catch in an abalone shell. If I have loose sage, I put the leaves in the shell to burn. I use a large feather to move the smoke from the sage to clean the areas and people, letting the aromatic and cleansing smoke reach the ceiling, floors, and each corner of the room. I then do the same to any person entering into the protected space. I take them outside and wave the sage so that the smoke circles and swirls around the entire person. I have them stand still with their feet apart and their arms out to the sides. I wave the smoke stick down and around each arm, around their hands, up and down the center line and the throat, around their head, and down and around their legs. I have them lift their feet and carefully swirl the smoke under each foot. I then tell them to turn around and do the same to their back side as well. Sometimes I will lightly slap the smudge stick to get more smoke into a certain area.

Mirrors: Mirrors are incredible deflectors. When facilitating someone else's healing, point a mirror away from your chest to protect you from any unwanted energy coming at you. You can either imagine a mirror or wear a small one, either will work.

The White Cloak: Imagine yourself stepping into a white light cloak all around you as you enter the space to work on someone. While you must always keep your person protected, you also must keep yourself protected. You don't know what that person will be bringing into a session, and you do not need to absorb it. Stay inside your white light cloak at all times.

Crystals and Pendants: Wearing stones will also help protect you, and people commonly buy necklaces specifically for protection or to increase energy. An easy one to start with is a simple clear quartz, which helps transmute energies and keep you protected. Smoky quartz helps dispel negative energy. A lot of energy workers will be sure to have a smoky quartz on them somewhere if not around the neck. Wearing a rose quartz near your heart is wonderfully blissful, as it is a stone of unconditional love. I like to use apophyllite stones at the head and foot of my table to keep my energy and the recipient's energy separate. Having two of these stones is very important to me while engaging in this work. They are not nearly as easy to find as most of the stones. The other stone I prefer to have in twos (and equally difficult to find) is the Girasol opal. This is the stone of truth telling. When people hold one in each hand, things come out of them that they would never consciously plan to reveal. I use these when I need someone to get really specific and deeply honest with themselves. Black tourmaline is the powerful protector stone and might be useful if you need a little extra help there. Jet is also a stone for protection, especially against your own personal fears. When I was in the throes of anxiety, you would likely find photos of me with this necklace on. I still have it hanging in the corner of the children's bedrooms to keep the bad dreams or negative energy out of their space. There are many books on crystals out there; I recommend a basic one to get started. Or, you can simply find crystals that resonate with you and go from there.

Sea Salt: This humble ingredient is an excellent protector and energy cleanser. I keep a bowl of sea salt in my practice room at all times. I rub a pinch between my hands so that I can clear myself of the energy of the person I've just been treating. You can place salt in any room to help protect the space and to help clear it of negative energy. Sprinkle it on any person (including yourself!) to help purify their energies. To strengthen the effect, mix the salt with holy water and sprinkle it down the spine, the crown of the head, or on the palms of the hands or soles of the feet. Sea salt is also wonderful for a detox bath to help release impurities from the body.

Psychic Protection Setup

Clean the space you intend to protect. In one corner, place a small glass bowl of sea salt (earth element). Then set a glass bowl of water (water element, preferably holy water or water you have prayed over and set intentions into) in the next. For the third corner, place one burning candle (fire element). Finally, in the last corner, burn one incense stick (air element). Although a Feng Shui practitioner would probably disagree, I've found that any corner is fine for any element. Even if people aren't sensitive to energy, you will find when you set up a room with this intention, it will be felt. It's a powerful way to keep the space energetically protected and clean.

Part V
The Spiritual Body

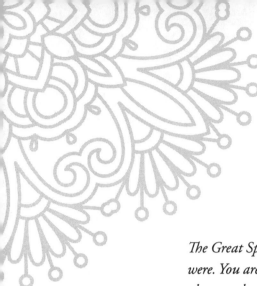

The Great Spirit is always with you. You are not alone. You never were. You are loved. You are protected. Open up to the deep spaces above and within. Listen to the wisdom of the Divine. Everyone is gifted and this includes YOU.

Chapter 12
Introduction to Spirit Work

Your spiritual body is referred to as many things: your soul, spirit, inner wisdom, inner physician, great spirit, or simply your god/goddess. The name is unimportant, so use what you feel comfortable with. This is our inherent connection to the source of all that is: God, the Universe, Great Spirit, the Divine. The name is not nearly as important as the connection itself. It is the part of ourselves that has the universal life force energy and what makes us consciously alive. I hope to help you connect with the Divine in a way that makes you feel safe, loved, comfortable, protected, and enhanced. There is something out there that is bigger than all of us; my goal is to help you find your way into to the spirit world in a way that resonates with you personally. If you choose to connect deeply and tap into this space, I believe it can alter the course of your life in some of the most profound ways. Personally speaking, I would be lost without my spirit team.

We all came from the other side, and we will return to the other side. Hopefully in this incarnation we strive to stay connected to the highest path of opportunities for our soul's growth. And it is within this space that each next right step along your ultimate journey is found. Spirit is the place I turned to each and every time during my recovery and especially during my child's recovery. Going to friends for guidance can make you spin your wheels with all the "you should try this" or "you should try that" advice. It's easy to get overwhelmed and drowned out in voices that are not your own, but there is no greater authority on your health and your life than the help and suggestions of Great Spirit. In saying this, however, I also understand that getting to the place where you feel connected and able to receive those messages can be tricky.

Connecting to Spirit through Loss

When faced with an incredible, life-shattering loss through death, many times we turn to mystics and mediums or communicators to help us to connect with the spirits of the departed. We desperately want to stay connected and know that our loved ones are still with us and comfortable on the other side. Likewise, if we've experienced tremendous loss not through death but through events like heartbreak or rejection and we want answers to help us understand, we can seek psychics and other spirit workers to help us make sense of it all. We've seen people on TV who can communicate with the other side, and I've been to many people who have helped me communicate with loved ones and also who have helped me develop my own skills. It is a very natural progression into learning to communicate with Spirit to first find people who already know how to do so. Some can also teach you how to do it for yourself. While there are some incredibly intuitive and gifted psychics, channelers, and mediums in this world, they get a bad rap because there are probably just as many or more frauds out there.

Cautions on Your Spiritual Journey

When we engage on a spiritual path, it's common to think everything is a sign and can thus read into signs way too much; we can go overboard on green lights and red flags. Recently on my radio show, I interviewed an Ayurvedic author and chef. I asked a lot of questions about different foods under different situations, and I remember she answered with, "Many times in Ayurveda, the answer is *it depends*." This wisdom also applies when we jump onto a spiritual path. There are definitely signs everywhere, but some can lead you on a wild goose chase. It may sound confusing, but not everything is the sign you are actually looking for. For this reason, you must be very careful when including other people on your spiritual path. I gave my power away time and again to mystics, psychics, healers, and so on. It's not that these guides do not have their place; I still visit them as needed to this day, but it can become too easy to use them for everything. I began to mute my own voice and my own intuition and instead gave these people the power to decide what would happen or appear next in my life. It was a long journey to find my own power within, but doing so has made all the difference. Now I use my trusted advisors for second confirmation instead of the actual decision-making process. Getting to the place where you can trust your own instincts and communications is difficult; it requires constant practice and trust. I'm going to break down for you who's who in spiritual communication to create a map you might need as you travel into this arena.

When it comes to seeking advice from others who work with the spirit realm, I hate to admit that for a long time I was completely addicted. I went to a lot of people before I ever trusted myself and my own ability to communicate. There are some masterfully gifted mediums, psychics, and channelers. There are also scammers, manipulators, and greedy thieves. When it comes to this kind of work, finding the right one comes first from word of mouth of someone you trust. Even then, upon meeting the spirit worker, you *must* trust your own feelings and instincts. If you are filling in too many blanks, answering questions for them, feeding them too much information, and so on, watch yourself—they may not be authentic. You may be overly eager and take away things that weren't in the session. Sit back, answer questions with only a little giveaway, and try to receive the information they offer neutrally. Most importantly, if someone's energy ever makes you feel uncomfortable or off, leave immediately. Remember that we are only working with the highest light for our healing; doing so should never make us feel uneasy or uncomfortable. After having a session you believed had value, sit with it. Take your time in making the decision to return. Anyone who tries to pressure you into another session does not have your highest good in mind.

Medium

A medium serves as a go-between for the spirit and human realms. They are able to communicate with spirit. I recommend seeing these people when you need to get some answers from a deceased loved one (including pets). When mediums make contact with the other side, they are generally fully conscious and present as they listen and interpret what the loved one needs you to know.

Channeling

A person who channels allows a spirit to use their body as a means of communication, like in the movie *Ghost* when Patrick Swayze's character stepped inside Whoopi Goldberg's character's body to communicate with Molly, his loved one (Demi Moore), but not nearly as animated. Spirits don't come in with a giant *whoosh!* that makes the channeler's hair fly back and their eyes dart open. That said, a channeler may visibly change when they are actually engaged in the channeling. They might close their eyes so as not to overwhelm, or they may keep their eyes open but no longer look the same. It's hard to describe, but when you find a good one it's a very unique experience, not a scary one.

One of the channelers I've worked with described the practice of channeling as moving to the back of the bus. She's still on the bus but has let someone else drive while she sits in the back. At any time, she could walk to the front of the bus and reclaim the driver's seat.

Channelers tend to open their bodies up to spirits who are not necessarily loved ones but rather Ascended Masters and other spirit guides coming from a higher light dimension. Many times, a departed loved one will not know how to work with a channeler, so a channeling session may not be ideal if you are trying to connect to a specific person. If you are trying to communicate with Spirit and receive messages but don't have a preconceived connection request, channeling can be a profound experience. Be sure to see someone who can maintain control of the situation. They need to be able to hold the space and only allow higher light sources through. If you find someone who may possess this gift but has not done any real work to hone or control it, look elsewhere for someone with more experience. I've been around people who like to open up to spirits only when drinking alcohol or under an influence; doing so in that state does not give them control over what enters. In fact, I've been in a situation where someone under the influence opened themselves up to any and all spirits. I immediately grabbed my keys and ran right out the door—I am not here to play around with things like this. Drugs or substances that dull the senses bring around darker energies. Do not play around in the spirit world.

Psychics

A psychic is someone you visit to gain insight into things ahead. The term "psychic" is interchangeable with "fortune-teller," and there are many levels of this kind of ability. When seeking out a psychic, your local metaphysical store is a great place to begin. Most owners have already tested and filtered through their psychics' abilities before hiring them. As well, many established metaphysical stores will offer intuitive development classes, which will help you make your way into the spirit world for communication purposes.

Palmistry

By reading the lines on a person's palms, a palm reader can give a lot of insight, seeing what has happened and what is destined to happen. My friend lost her boyfriend when she was twenty-five years old. He died very suddenly, and his death completely changed everything in our lives. My previous belief systems were challenged as he made contact with us several times within the following year. I went from being totally against the concept of past lives and "New Age stuff" to not being able to learn enough. How could I disbelieve a spirit sitting in front of me telling me what life was now like for him? He would wake me up at night to listen to him so I could tell my friend what he had to say. He would say, "You gotta wake up because you can see me and she can't. You can hear me and she can't!" I offer this story to say that whenever she went to a palm reader, she always knew if they were the real deal by whether they could pick up by reading her palm that she had a significant loss around the age of twenty-five. Most could see it easily and pick it up. If they did, she'd proceed with the reading. If they missed it, she would cut the reading short and move on.

Of course, not all of us have a cross on our palms in the center of the fate line like she did. It is worth noting that as major situations happen in our lives, our lines of the hands do change, though the lines on the right palm change more often than the lines on the left. Our palms are the maps to our soul contract: the left hand's lines are what Spirit gives you, and the right hand's lines are a reflection of what you do with it. I've only had a few people ever read me through my palms but they were spot on with it. One palm reader could actually identify my top four angels I always call in, and he was spot on with information from that point onward.

Palmistry is a highly sacred art that requires training either passed down within a family tradition or intense private study. It is an intuitive and very detailed practice. If you decide you want to see someone for a palm reading, check around your area and read reviews, or inquire with your local metaphysical bookstores for a recommendation. If you attend any spirit expos or psychic fairs, there is usually someone there who can do it well. In my experience, really extraordinary palm readers are not easy to find, and I don't tend to seek them out; they tend show up out of the blue when I need them.

Divination Tools

There are many ways people can connect into the spirit realm, and it's not always with deep meditation and inner guidance (though rest assured, we will be covering those methods too). Pendulums, rune stones, tarot, and oracle cards can be extremely insightful. I use these all the time to help me get an answer or perspective on whatever I'm concerned with at the moment. I think there are times during any healing journey where going to see someone who can help you identify and locate whatever can help you heal are the most valuable tools out there. This avenue can provide wonderful offerings. Much like the physical body section that covered who to see for what condition, navigating your way through psychics and readers is equally as daunting.

Even greater than finding someone who can throw rune stones, read cards, or dowse with a pendulum is learning how to do these things yourself. Ideally, you want to get to a place where if you are in doubt or need some quick answers, you can rely on some of your own abilities. It is important to note that I am by no means an expert on each divination tool; what's here is a compilation of research, not personal practice. Keep in mind that there is no one "best" divination tool. All have their place, and it's perfectly natural to be drawn to some methods over others.

Writing

A great many people write or journal for divination purposes … whether they realize that's what they are doing or not. This is a powerful way to tap into not just your own energy but also to communicate and open yourself to receive direct communication. Mediums or other spirit workers often keep a note pad with them when they are in the space of communication. They may or may not write coherently, as writing like this might be simply their way of getting their bodies into the space in which they are able to line up their vibration in order to connect. Writing clears the mind without effort to do so. Journaling and asking to hear your communication can be simpler than you may think. Asking questions on paper with the dominant hand and answering with the nondominant hand can help you get to your child brain for memory retrieval. When writing to spirits directly— be it your angels, spirit guide/s, God/Goddess—be sure to list them by name. Then as you write your thoughts or questions, either again change hands, or keep using your dominant hand and begin to write answers that you feel might be coming through. When you are new to this way of connecting, you can feel like you are just making up answers in your head. More times than not, this is not the case. You are tapping in and hearing the information. They just deliver it so softly that it takes us a while to understand that this is how the communication can go.

Automatic Writing: Channeled writing or psychography is a way of writing that directly channels through you from the spirit realm. You are not consciously aware all the time of the things you write; instead you are opening yourself up to Spirit to channel through you. This type of writing is much like energy work; you clear yourself as a channel and Spirit guides your hands.

Journal Prompts: Here you are journaling but answering a set of questions. You are ascertaining your own views. Example: "Let's write about depression. How do I feel about my depression? What is causing my depression?" Prompts are good for when you don't know what you want to write but could answer a direct question at length. They can also help you get started if you are completely new to journaling. As for finding prompts, they can be found all over the place these days, and about any topic—anxiety, courage, depression—any subject you can think of has journal prompts available. You can also write your own journal prompts on any subject. Because prompts are like a springboard to get you into the writing process, they can be an excellent way of creating your own self-help.

Free-form Writing: In this style of journaling, you simply start writing about absolutely anything and see where it goes. Even without a set starting point, you will inevitably find something in your writing that you didn't expect you'd talk about. Free-form writing can be a great indicator of where your mind is in a process. Do you notice patterns? A good way to get started is to make it a goal to at least fill up an entire page. Then use the writing to help you intuit what is really going on within the deeper layers of your mind. It will look random at first, but then you will be led deeper into what is really going on inside.

Tarot

The classic tarot deck has seventy-eight cards with a major and minor arcana. The major arcana is twenty-one cards and represents the hero's journey from being the fool to becoming wise. The four suits of the minor arcana correspond to the four elements of earth, air, fire, and water: cups (emotions/water), wands (will/fire), swords (thought/air), and pentacles (physical/earth).

There are a lot of ways tarot can be used, though it is best used as a tool for self-exploration. Most modern readers use tarot as a tool to integrate the conscious and subconscious minds. Some pull tarot cards to receive insight about any given situation. You can also use it to discern the deeply secretive driving forces that you or someone else with an attachment might be concealing. Tarot is extremely accurate for situations as they currently stand, but understand that it is only accurate for that exact moment in time. Situations can change, and therefore a new reading might be necessary.

When working with a tarot reader, here are some things to look for:

1. Readers do not predict the future; they show you possibilities.
2. A standard tarot reader uses the cards to discern what is happening in the present. Cards can present insight, in other words "If you continue on the path you are on, this is what is likely to occur. If you choose this other way, *this* is likely to occur." Keep in mind that other people can change situations. Tarot offers guided clarity only into what is happening exactly right now.
3. Some people are able to use the tarot deck to provide guidance for the future and fortune telling, but not all readers are skilled at this.

When looking for a reader, trust word of mouth more than ratings. Ask people you trust who they see, and above all, trust your gut. If you see someone for a reading but don't feel as though they are well versed or very skilled, keep looking. There are a ton of readers out there and just as many tarot decks with varying themes. Try to find readers who know their decks well and feel in alignment with your energy.

Oracle Decks

Unlike the tarot, which has a foundation of math and science (they are set out in a mathematical, systematic pattern), oracle cards are more intuitive and less systematic. There are many different variations of oracle cards, and basically anyone can use them. Compared to the tarot, they are much more user friendly and require less study and training to be effective. I have several different decks of cards and choose a deck according to whatever information I am trying to find. The easiest way to get started using oracle cards is to shuffle them and fan them out face down. Close your eyes, get quiet, and ask a question. Wherever your hand is drawn, pull that card. While tarot cards have different meanings depending on their orientation (tarot cards have different meanings depending on of the cards are right side up or upside down, i.e., reversals), oracle cards tend not to have rules regarding card placement (that said, read your particular deck to see if it has any rules). Whatever card you have drawn will serve as a message and tool to give insight. You can also pull cards according to the various spreads usually offered in the booklet that comes with the deck. These spreads (usually they aren't too complicated) allow for deeper information and possible alternative meaning. If you don't want to get into spreads, you can also pull three cards and lay them side by side. The card on the left signifies what occurred in the past, the center card is a message for the present, and the card on the right shows what is ahead for you.

Rune Stones

Rune stones are a set of stones that have a specific image or glyph on each one. It is possible to find stones with personalized or other phonetic alphabets, but they are not the norm. The stones are usually accompanied by a book or a chart that outlines the name of each rune and its meaning. There are a few ways to work with rune stones. Usually a person will place the stones in a bowl or a bag and then draw runes without looking or toss all the stones onto a cloth. There are several rules when it comes to rune stone reading, and etiquette varies from cultural practice to cultural practice and from reader to reader.

Runes are commonly considered a practice for yourself, and it's easy to learn to read on your own. If you need a singular answer to a particular situation, runes are a great bet, as they can be far more direct than tarot or oracle cards. That said, they can also be harsh because they cut right to the chase!

Pendulums

The pendulum is used for dowsing and moves based on the energy it receives through your body. When you use a pendulum, you become the oracle. It is an indicator of the energy that is flowing through your body at that particular moment. It's a guiding mark to what you are asking. The best way to start with a pendulum is to ask it questions that you already know the truth of the answer. Make sure that the *yes* and *no* match what is true.

Check it on a question that definitely has a right and wrong answer, such as your name. Ask the pendulum out loud, "Is my name _____?" and see if it swings to a *yes* or *no*. If it swings *yes*, you can use the pendulum as your guide because it is in alignment with your energy for questioning.

Pendulums are my favorite divination tool; I use them all the time. While different people have different ways of working with a pendulum, there are a few tips that cover many bases. Be sure to clear your space and ask only the highest light to work with you. Also either have your elbow flat as you hold the end of the chain or string between your fingers or hold your hand and arm up and allow the pendulum to dangle. And before you begin with learning the pendulum's directions, you must clear your space, state your intentions, and let the pendulum itself know which directions are *yes*, *no*, *maybe*, and *ask again*. I prefer to do up and down for *yes* and side to side for *no*. If it goes in a circle or in a diagonal, I know the answer is not yet decided, I need to ask again at another time, or ask in another way. Some people do not use up and down as *yes*, but use circling one direction for *yes* and another direction for *no*. There is not a right or wrong way; it's all about clarity and intention.

The questions you ask a pendulum are yes/no questions, and they must be framed to have a *yes* or *no* answer. You can't receive a complicated answer or even one that requires explanation, so you must be careful how you ask. Even if you follow these rules and ask the right questions, pendulum work can be tricky. Your mind can alter the direction of the answers. If you find yourself asking things with an answer you are hoping or pushing for, it's hard to get a proper read. If I ask a question such as "Will my book proposal be picked up?" while at the same time constantly wishing "Say yes, say yes," it's very tough to get an honest read. In situations like this, it's difficult but best to clear our minds, put the pendulum down, and ask again later.

Chapter 13
Gathering Your Spirit Team

This chapter explores various spirit masters and deities. If you are not interested in learning anything more than the ones you know already, feel free to skip this chapter without pressure or guilt.

There are a lot of spirit helpers, angels and ascended masters in the Universe. Learning about them and getting to know them can be incredibly helpful as you open up to a wider way of working with the spirit realm. This is only offered as a guide for you to learn your own way in working with the highest light masters. After clearing the space and setting my intentions, I call on God first. Use whatever name that means to you. As I offer the lists below notice if you feel pulled to any name or energy. From there, I urge you to further study them so that you can work with them to the fullest extent.

- Jesus: Christian (Part of the Trinity: Father, Son, and Holy Spirit)
- Mary: Christian (Virgin Mother of Christ)
- Moses: Jewish
- Allah: Muslim
- Muhammad: Muslim
- Buddha: Buddhist
- Quan Yin: Taoist
- Brahma/Shiva/Vishnu: (Hindu Trinity)
- White Buffalo Calf Woman: Lakota
- Gura Nanak: Sikh
- Bahá'u'lláh: Bahá'í

Ascended Masters

An Ascended Master is someone who, in life, was a great spiritual teacher or healer and is now in the spirit realm. These people lived extraordinary lives and served a great number of people. We cannot list every Ascended Master, but what follows is a basic foundation:

- Jesus: Considered the son of God in the Christian tradition.
- Mary: The Virgin Mother of Christ in the Christian tradition.
- Mary Magdalene: The most well-known woman follower of Jesus.
- Melchizedek: Associated with the Archangel Michael and Jesus in many texts. He helps with the spiritual laws of attraction. He is also an Old Testament priest and the first one to proclaim the coming of the Messiah.
- Paramahansa Yogananda: Author of *Autobiography of a Yogi*. Well known in aiding yoga practitioners on their spiritual path.
- El Morya: Considered one of the Ancient Masters of Theosophy. Helps to keep your energy clean of any darkness.
- St. Germain: Not a Catholic saint, but a German count considered to be one of the world's greatest philosophers. St. Germain can help bring about miracles in a very short time period.
- St. Francis of Assisi: Aids in communication and comfort to animals.
- Buddha (Siddhartha Gautama Buddha at birth): Became enlightened while sitting under the bodhi tree. Believes in the end of suffering through nonattachment.
- Quan Yin: Taoist and Buddhist goddess of mercy and receiver of all prayers.
- Krishna: Hindu god of compassion and wisdom. It is one of Krishna's dialogues that created the *Bhagavad-Gita*, one of Hinduism's sacred texts.
- Lakshmi: Hindu goddess of prosperity and wealth.
- Kali: Hindu goddess of fury. She can help clear the negative energy away and fiercely protect you.
- Ganesha: Hindu god who clears the path for healing. Often prayed to first.
- White Buffalo Calf Woman: Lakota sacred woman, responsible for bringing forth the sacred pipe.

- Moses: A prophet of great courage. Most associated with the parting of the Red Sea and delivering the Jews to the promised land. Helps with courage.
- Babaji: A renowned yogi, known as the "deathless avatar."
- Green Man: A Pagan deity, considered the face of nature and helps with fertility of crops.
- Serapis: Greco-Egyptian god of ascension.

The Hindu trinity:

- Vishnu: The preserver
- Shiva: The destroyer
- Brahma: The creator

Spirit Guides

A spirit guide is a spirit who is still in the incarnation cycle. You and the spirit made an agreement before you entered your life, that they will guide you along your entire path for this incarnation and that you will do the same for them in the future. It is not possible to make this agreement with someone who was alive with you who then passed on. Of course, the soul of your deceased loved one is with you and will provide guidance. However, your loved one is not your primary spirit guide because the contract was made before you entered life and will still be with you beyond this life. Once you reenter the incarnation cycle, you will do the same for your spirit guide. You will guide them throughout their life. A spirit guide is someone you are very close to on a soul level.

Often when we think our subconscious is speaking, it is in fact our spirit guide. Have you ever been driving down the road and decide to take a different route for no good reason? Maybe something in the back of your mind said not to, but you did it anyway and then found out you really should have gone the original way. You say to yourself, "I *knew* I should've gone the other way." Well that was your spirit guide you ignored! Your guide was speaking to you. Sometimes we listen and sometimes we don't … but most of the time we wish we did. Don't beat yourself up; this is all part of the pact. Spirit guides know they are going to be frustrated with us because our natural reaction is to brush them off as not real. Too many of us think we don't have the gift to hear Spirit, but we actually hear Spirit all the time—we just don't know the difference. Imagine that little birdie sitting on your shoulder right by your ear, trying to get through to you. They scream, they yell, they jump up and down … and we hear nothing. Or we do hear it but just as quickly dismiss what we heard. After all, we don't like to buy into the crazy. Maybe we should listen to the crazy a little more often, as it can help us bypass a lot of crap! When you think about the red flags people mention all the time, who do you think that is that makes us see them? Is it our subconscious or is it our guide? Some say they are one in the same.

Angels

If there's one thing I love about angels, it's that all the major religions embrace their presence.[31] While the value placed on these celestial beings varies widely, they all have mention as servants of the Divine. I love angels so much and ask for their assistance every single day of my life. I may ask certain angels to watch over my children while they are at school, watch over us as we travel, or help me when seeking clarity. I believe we all at the very least are born with a guardian angel who stays with us through our life. Other angels might come and go as needed, but our guardian is always there. So many people have varying opinions on the physical nature of angels: whether they are male/female, have wings, and so on. One of my favorite stories is from when I attended a talk given by psychic and author Sylvia Brown. She said she had given another big talk elsewhere where she said that angels don't really look the way we envision them, telling the whole crowd that angels don't really have wings. That same night, she woke in the middle of the night to get a glass of water. She went down to her kitchen, and what do you suppose appeared before her but a giant angel with wings that spanned beyond the kitchen doorway? She said she looked up at the angel and said: "Damn! You *do* have wings," and went back to bed.

As for my own angel encounters, they happened after the first time I ever attended a yoga class back in the 1990s. At the end of the class, the teacher had us lie down for *savasana*, or corpse pose. In it, you lie as still as you can while the teacher takes you through a guided meditation to calm the body and mind. This relaxation technique also allows the muscles to absorb the practice that had just occurred into memory. Before having us come out of meditation, he had us reach our arms overhead and open our palms. He came by and put a few drops of the most heavenly scented oil blend onto our palms. We were

---

31. Encyclopedia Britannica, "Varieties of Angels and Demons in the Religions of The World," https://www
.britannica.com/topic/angel-religion/Varieties-of-angels-and-demons-in-the-religions-of-the-world.

to rub our hands together and then smell the oil before opening our eyes. The blend had lavender, ylang-ylang, lily of the valley, and almond oil. That night after yoga, I went to bed and woke to three giant light beings in the corner of my room—one blue, one yellow, and one green. They expanded from the floor up the wall and onto the ceiling. The light was bright but translucent at the same time. One by one, they came up from behind me and wrapped themselves around me, turned to the left and then disappeared. On the third and final one, I managed to open my eyes fully. It was still there, as bright as I saw it in my mind's eye. I instantly knew that this was my first real angel encounter.

Many people have their own stories of angel encounters. If you haven't had one, all you need to do is begin to connect to the angels and create a line of communication and connection between them and yourself. The more you make yourself open, the more they can get through to you. I went back to that yoga teacher and asked to purchase that exact bottle of oil hoping for continued connections. I never was able to recreate such an experience. It is something I will treasure always.

There are said to be nine levels of angels, divided into three different triads. As you read this section, if a certain level or name of an angel resonates with you, use it as a starting point for connecting to them. Ask your angels for guidance or to reveal themselves to you in whatever way feels comfortable and safe to you both. You can ask for them to come to you in your dreams, through shiny objects like pennies and dimes on the street, in finding feathers, or through prayer or other thoughts and impressions in your mind.

First Triad: Seraphim, Cherubim, Throne

The seraphim are the first and highest level of the first triad, said to be the closest to God. This order of angelic servants supposedly appears with six wings and four heads. They are beings of pure light who keep darkness away from divinity. They shine so bright that humans are unlikely to see them.

The second level of angels in the first triad are the cherubim. These are angels of harmony and wisdom, of boundless love and knowledge, and guardians of the temples. These are what we see in paintings and sculptures: little potbellied angels, beautiful, and childlike.

Third are the throne angels. These are considered many-eyed angels who govern justice and will as well as planetary issues. These angels create and send positive energy.

Second Triad: Dominions, Virtues, Powers

The first of the second triad of angels are the dominions. These are Divine leaders who help with intuition and wisdom as well as mediation and arbitration—especially when leaders of church and state are unable to agree on the best outcome. I wonder, are we able hear them? Are we listening?

Second in the second triad are the virtues, who are understood to be the angels of miracles. They send healing energy to the Universe and gravitate toward the light workers on our planet.

Last in the second triad are the powers, the angels of space and form. These angels have helped along the way with world religions and are the keepers of human history. They are perfect to call on for protection.

Third Triad: Principalities, Archangels, Angels

The third triad of angels is considered the lowest of the choirs, which means that they are the closest to our human realm of existence.

The first of these are the principalities. These are the angels of time who also guard continents, countries, and cities. They are protectors of politics and religion and they channel positive energy to help with global reform. I think it would be in our best interest to help introduce more people to this group.

Next are my personal favorites, the archangels. These angels are said to enjoy human contact, which is probably why these are the angels we interact with most often. These beautiful beings belong to several levels in the hierarchy of the angelic realm. I feel the most kinship with these angels. Here are some of their names and their associations.

Note: This list does not include every single archangel, but it is a great place start. The first four are who I always call on first, followed by the rest.

- Michael: The protector. With his violet-blue flame sword, Michael protects us from evil.
- Raphael: Healing angel, considered God's medicine angel.
- Gabriel: The angel who forecasted the coming of Christ and helped write the Koran. Gabriel infuses us with creativity and helps with information.
- Uriel: Aids in grounding, known as the angel of wisdom.
- Jophiel: Helps with peace, joy, and nature.

- Azrael: Aids in the dying process.
- Ariel: Rules over animals and nature.
- Sandalphon: Helps you expand your spiritual gifts.
- Metatron: Considered the record keeper. Aids in organization and record-keeping. Metatron is also known to work with children, especially those with sensory issues and special needs.
- Chamuel: Helps put us on our best career path. Chamuel also helps us locate lost things such as keys. If a pet or a person become lost, call on Archangel Chamuel for assistance.

The last group of the final triad (though certainly not the least important) is the one closest to us. These are simply called the angels, the ones we know best. These beautiful light protectors and messengers are our guardian angels. These oversee the plants, the trees, the animals, the minerals, and us humans. These are the beings who help us transition from birth to death. They are very playful and the easiest for us to communicate with, but they will not usually intervene. They are with us and looking out for our best interest; sometimes we hear their guidance, sometimes we do not.

If you do not currently work with the angels, I would love to put it out there and ask you to try it. Do your own testing to see if you can feel their presence. Be open to communication and ask them to give you confirmation that they are with you. Angels are always there for guidance and comfort, and it's easiest to feel them once you open the pathways of communication. Feeling their presence is a two-way street: be open to receive their guidance and support and remember the truth—you are never alone. Sometimes it's really hard to believe and remember that the angels are always with us, especially when we find ourselves in a low place. Trust that these beautiful, loving guides are eager to assist and walk with you. They are only waiting to be invited.

Chapter 14

Getting Connected

There are many ways in which we might feel the presence of a loved one or a spiritual presence; it might be through sight, sounds, a feeling, a song, a scent, or dreams. Once we can pinpoint our best way of connecting with the energies around us, it opens up an avenue for deeper study of our communication abilities and styles.

The Four Clairs

It is important that we learn the best ways that we are able to communicate with the spirit realm, and our exploration of the four clairs in this chapter will show you how to tap in and find out yours. Gaining an understanding into these areas and how you best relate can very much improve the way that you work with energy. Once you realize how you are able to receive messages most clearly, you can begin to work within that specific skill to hone your spirit game, which will in turn help you as you work with your team more effectively. As you read through the following sections, try not to get attached to a specific clair; none of us get to choose the way we connect. Instead, sit with each and find out how it happens for you. For example, a lot of people out there want to be able to see spirit; after all, seeing is believing. But when some people discover they do not have that gift, they decide that they don't have any gifts at all. If this is the case for you, don't despair—your gift might be in clear knowing (clairsentience), not clear seeing (clairvoyance). And even if your gift is clear seeing, maybe you've kept it hidden because people might think you are crazy. Go through these gifts and then sit with each of them. Whichever one makes you go back to reread is likely your strongest one. Learn about the ways in which you are able to perceive messages.

Clear your mind of preconceived notions. Once you get situated and comfortable with the avenue of your gifts, let it become your starting point for communication.

1. Clairaudience: Clear listening, or the ability to hear sounds others may not be able to hear. You can hear Spirit whispering in your ear. Sometimes we hear things and turn around. We wonder who was speaking to us, only to find no one there. People with this gift need to keep their ears open and know that they are not crazy. I personally am extremely clairaudient; in most cases, messages come to me in the form of music. I hear different songs when I'm with different people, more so if my hands are on them. I will literally hear words to a song that is describing where someone is in their current space. As we work together, the songs change (almost like the dial on a radio being turned) and I hear different sounds or lyrics. I remember an interview with Sting one time where he reported that whenever he met people, he could hear different instruments in his head. It was how he identified people's energy and received an impression of them.

2. Clairvoyance: Clear vision, or the ability to actually see Spirit. Many people who can see Spirit speak of being able to see it in their mind's eye rather than the spirit actually standing in front of them (although some highly advanced people can see them in this manner). Children are naturally clairvoyant—have you ever seen a child look around a room and wonder what they see? They see angels and guides everywhere. Unlike us, they don't know that it's not "normal," To them, it is completely natural—as it should be (until we take it away from them)!

3. Claircognizance: The ability of clear knowing, or to "just know" things without asking why. I believe mothers are very good at this, mostly with their children, but anyone could just as easily have this ability with their Spirit Team. If you know something in your gut, trust it. Personally, I always try to trust my gut, but getting there took a really long time and a lot of concentrated effort.

4. Clairsentience: Clear feeling. People who have this ability are generally referred to as empaths, as they can sense energies. Clairsentient people can hold an object and sense the energy, events, or a person's energy associated with the object, a practice known as psychometry. If you feel something coming, positive or negative, this is you tapping into this ability. When you're around somebody and can

feel their pain, that is you tapping into the ability. Many people who work in the healthcare industry (nurses, therapists, energy workers, and so on) are highly intuitive, empathic people who often practice this gift. Along with claircognizance and clairaudience, clairsentience are my strongest gifts. I can tap into and feel all sorts of things, and I know what I know when I feel it. I've learned to always trust it. I don't want to say I'm always right with my psychic hits and messages, but I do believe that my spirit helpers don't steer me wrong.

Quieting the Body

A vital practice of spiritual communication is knowing how to "quiet" yourself effectively. Sometimes we refer to this as being still or centering ourselves, or a kind of meditation. Whether you practice centering prayer, meditate, or just enjoy quiet time spent outside, learning how to effectively get still inside yourself is the very best way to get into a space that allows for communication with your soul self.

Quieting the body is different from quieting the mind. To quiet the body means coming into a place where your physical body can be without any movement. This is a situation in which the mind and body can help one another; when both are in unison in a soft, relaxing space, meditation becomes something of a practice and communication can become more likely. For this section, we will focus on calming the body first. If it's easier for you to do this while lying down, start there. If you can do this while sitting cross-legged with a straight spine and open palms, even better. The manner in which you are positioned is not vital to the process, but it is part of the setting of intention. Some people can do it best while standing but relaxed. No matter how you do it, the moment you begin to quiet down, you will notice that your body often has a tough time getting comfortable. Sensations begin to amplify. The tag in your shirt, the sensation of your hair, any pains that have been lurking—they all come up in a multitude of ways when you attempt to be still. This is perfectly normal and happens to the best of us. The goal is to sit with those irritations long enough to relax and let go. Acknowledge the annoyance's existence and then let it pass. Remember that being patient with this process aids in expanding the practice, and getting frustrated with yourself will do the opposite. No matter your body position for quieting yourself, know that you can achieve stillness. You will wait out the scratches, itches, weird sensations, and so on. Eventually you will win the body over either through time spent or using the mind to detach from physical annoyances. Both can get you to where you want to be, but you must practice. Keep coming back to your practice of centering and stilling the body. Do your practice in small increments, daily for best results.

Quieting the Mind

Learning to quiet the mind is different from learning to still the physical body. The mind becomes explosive when you try to come to a central point of focus and awareness. The monkey mind becomes loud and aggressive and will try anything to make you pay attention to it. Maybe you begin to compile a list of all the things you "need" to think about; all the items that need to be on your shopping list are of *prime* importance for some reason, now that you are trying to be quiet. When learning how to let the mind get to a still point, sometimes you have to take another route to get there. As you know from reading this book, I tend to offer up the backdoor routes to our desired destination when the straightforward ways don't work. When the mind gets wired and fired, the best thing to do is ask for those thoughts to come in without reservation. Invite it all in instead of fighting against it. Now the trick is to take a step back from it and watch it all dance. You are no longer attached to your thoughts but are present for each one that comes in. You aren't ignoring the thoughts, nor are you condemning them with a "Shh! Quiet!" mentality either. You are simply opening up to whatever comes through without attachment.

If you own dogs, maybe you've been told or have learned that if you yell at them when they are already barking, they think you are joining them and get louder. In other words, you are playing into a hyped-up energy that is already there. But if you refrain from yelling at your dog and take the calm approach to counterbalance the frenzy, they will likely follow your lead. It's the same here: if you stay long enough with your monkey mind, it will tire itself out and take a nap. At worst, you will also tire out and take a nap as you wait for the mind to calm—a perfectly wonderful way to start with centering, quieting, and meditation as well. There is not a set of hard, fast rules on how to get yourself to quiet down. It only matters that you figure it out in the end. If you fall asleep, you've let yourself go enough to relax into a slumber. It's certainly not a bad thing, though you should try not to let it become a habit. Meditation is a very specific time set out to get quiet and begin a practice of connecting yourself into the rhythm and flow of the Universe.

⌘ Practice: Quieting the Body and Mind

Here you will use your body to help your mind calm and your mind to help your body calm. Both can work in unison to get you to where you want to be once you learn how to work within yourself. Begin by calming down the physical body. There are a few ways to do this depending if your goal is to be standing, sitting, or lying down. I will take you through the various ways to place your body to get into a comfortable position that can help make it easier to receive information that might come through. Once we've learned the best physical body ways to get calm and quiet, we'll add the mental piece that can go with any of the physical positions.

Option 1: Lying down: Lie down comfortably on your back in a place where you can unplug from the outside world. This could be in your bed or the floor. If you want to, place pillows under your knees. Bring the legs about 45 degrees out from the center line of the body and allow the feet to fall out to each side comfortably. Gently tuck the low back under and unroll the spine onto the surface beneath you. Bring the arms 45 degrees from the body and open the palms to face up to the sky. Slightly tuck your chin in but not down. This allows the base of the skull to lie comfortably against the surface beneath. Begin by taking a breath in and holding the breath as you tighten your feet, pointing your toes and lifting your legs one inch off the ground for just a moment. Exhale and drop the legs. Inhale and hold your breath as you lift your bottom and lower back off the floor and then exhale and relax and again lower the body and tuck the pelvis under. Inhale and lift your chest and upper back off the floor. Exhale and lower the back down and allow your spine to unroll itself onto the floor beneath. Inhale and lift your arms one inch off the ground, make a tight fist, then stretch your fingers out as wide as you can before you exhale and drop the arms back down. Inhale and lift your shoulders up to your ears and exhale and lower the shoulders back down. Gently turn your head so that one ear is on the floor. Slowly turn your head so that the other ear is to the floor. Lastly, inhale and hold the breath as you tighten all of the muscles on your face. Keep squeezing the jaws shut and the eyes closed tight. Exhale and open your eyes as wide as you can. Open your mouth as wide as you can. Stick your tongue out and exhale an audible roaring sound (this is the lion pose). Gently close your eyes and relax your jaws and allow your whole physical body to relax into itself. Notice your breath getting longer and deeper but quieter with its sound. Breathe and allow the energetic circulation to move throughout your entire body with each breath in and out.

Option 2: Sitting up in a chair: Put your feet flat with your back to the back of the chair. Keep your spine straight and chin slightly tucked in but not down. Your palms should face up, resting on your lap or in prayer position. It's a little bit more difficult in this position to work through the body tightening and relaxing the way you would lying down. When sitting, the relaxation is done better with the mind and breath coming together. For this practice, you must rely on auto suggestion to calm the body through the mind. You can think of your body part and ask it to relax.

Repeat:

• Relax my feet—my feet are relaxed.

• Relax my ankles, shins, and knees—my ankles, shins, and knees are relaxed.

• Relax my entire legs—my entire legs are relaxed.

• Relax my buttocks, pelvis, lower back, middle back, ribs, stomach, and intestines—my entire lower body is relaxed.

• Relax my chest and upper back—my chest and back are relaxed.

• Relax my shoulders, arms, and hands—my shoulders, arms, and hands are relaxed.

• Relax my neck and throat—my neck and throat are relaxed.

• Relax my head and scalp—my head and scalp are relaxed.

• Relax my face and ears—my face and ears are relaxed.

• Relax my entire body—my entire body is relaxed.

Option 3: Seated meditation: This is the most widely used meditation position. There are many reasons for this; however, I cannot say exactly why that is. My guess is because if sitting properly with good posture, the spine (as well as the energetic spine, the sushumna) can be fully opened and allows access into the mind and spirit with greater ease. In this position, it is more likely that you can open all of the chakras and experience the opening of the Kundalini Shakti.

The physical, energetic, emotional, and spiritual bodies all come together with a very strong conviction through this intention of proper body position and hand position. Place the palms facing up to receive the energy or with prayer hands to connect you into that cosmic energy. We sit legs crossed, either one in front of the other, one on top of the other, or in full lotus (where both legs are crossed and both feet rest up around the hip pockets of the legs). Try to avoid sitting cross-legged as you might naturally do it; one leg should be resting all the way over the other leg like a stacked wall rather than one foot blocking the energy of the other. Remember, energy moves throughout all of our limbs. We want to do all that we can to prevent ourselves from blocking any flow of the moving energy.

Option 4: Standing meditation: In practices of tai chi and qi gong, we use standing rather than seated meditation. We don't want to fully bend or block any part of the energy body. Stand with the feet flat and barefoot (preferably outside on the natural earth's surface). The feet should be shoulder width apart. The shoulders are slightly rounded. The crown of the head is directly facing the heavens without lifting the chin up. The chin is slightly tucked in, but not down. The tip of the tongue rests against the roof of the mouth behind the two front teeth and slightly back just at the mountain about an inch behind the two front teeth. The jaws are separated slightly in the mouth, and the top and bottom teeth are not touching. The hands can fall to your sides. The low back is slightly rounded and tucked under. Extend in your mind the tailbone as a real tail that goes all the way into the earth. The feet and tailbone tail make up the three points of balance for your body.

The knees are soft but not bent. Nothing is locked out—arms, legs, ankles, wrists; no locking or stiffness. Every joint and meridian line in your body is unobstructed, soft, and heavy. Try to allow all thoughts to come in until you can get to a space where you can empty them. Notice that the thoughts run straight through without any attachment until they filter out into a void of nothingness. You simply are one with heaven and earth. Freedom, healing, flow of energy is all that lives in this moment of peace, clarity, and unity with nature.

Hand Positioning

Hands are very much conductors of energy and can connect us to the quiet place in the body, in union with the mind. When we put the palms together at the chest in prayer position, we recognize that touching in that way produces something much deeper and profound. Putting your hands into prayer position is a universal hand mudra. There are also many other ways in which the hands conduct our connections, such as connecting the mudra of finger and thumb together while resting the hands on our knees. We see this in yoga and meditation practices while people sitting cross-legged or in full lotus position. There are many hand mudras where the various fingers represent different connections and movements, but rather than getting overly technical with hand positions, what we need to know is that any mudra is a conversation and connection between yourself and spirit. It's an intention that decrees something like: "I am about to engage in a meditation or spiritual practice. I will connect these fingers and close my eyes and sit quietly in order to ask that my practice be accompanied by the great spirits as I connect."

Clear the Mind

Once you have found your ideal position that will allow your body to get still, you can move into the mind for clearing. Begin by gathering your thoughts. Try to move those thoughts into a box with a tight lid and gently scoot them to the side of your mind and out of sight. We simply want to turn off the chatter. It is in the quieting of ourselves that communication is able to take place. The demands we would place on Spirit to have to yell and scream over our own wild mind is silly. They won't do it. They shouldn't have to do it. Create a space in which they can enter. Always first set your intentions with a prayer that only the highest light may enter.

⌘ Practice: The Funnel Slide

When the thoughts in your head become too chaotic, turn them around and let them slide down. Imagine a huge funnel slide that goes down to the ground. When the thoughts come flooding in or you feel your body reacting to the heightened energy, let the thoughts come into your head freely. Don't fight any of the feelings or thoughts—invite them in. Bring them all in and put them all on the slide: from the top of your head, watch those thoughts swirling down and around your body, out through your feet so that when it's done, it's done. You now leave them behind you. Once all the junky vibrations have emptied out and settled themselves, that's when you can slow down. Take the rest and fill yourself back up with positive dialogue and self-love.

Centering

If prayer is the act of talking to a higher source and meditation is listening to your higher source, then centering is something in between. When centering, you are not talking, nor may you be in a full space where you are able to listen. You are simply present and calm—centered. For the purpose of calming and quieting the mind, we turn away from prayer because the goal here is to become completely still and silent. We enter into a place where there is nothing but you and your energy. In this practice, you quiet yourself enough to be welcomed to enter cosmic consciousness, which may be thought of as an entirely different world of energy and movement someplace just above you.

By getting clear and quiet, you can enter into the cosmic flow where time and space cease to exist. It's always there, flowing and available, but you must be able to elevate your own consciousness in order to get yourself to this space. Anytime you choose to connect, you have to go deep within yourself in order to raise your vibration. Any chatter, doubting, or questioning will bring you back down into your body and in this plane. Whenever you rise up and enter this space, remember the practice and how it felt. As you practice more, you will be able to reach this higher vibration with greater confidence and ease.

✿ PRACTICE: CONNECT

Envision the Divine Spirit directly around your face and crown. Feel the energy collect around you. With eyes closed, begin to intermingle your breath with that of the Universe. Your exhale becomes the God/Goddess's inhale. The God/Goddess then exhales onto you as you inhale and take it in. It becomes an exchange, breath from one to the other. Keep your eyes closed, and don't get overly excited when you really begin to feel the exchange. The God/Goddess breathes out and you breathe it in. You breathe it out and they breathe it in. Continue for as long as you are able to be present and calm. Notice how your own energy expands with this practice.

You are in a place where your own vibration is raised so high that it is no longer in the physical realm of existence. This is not the time to observe your own thoughts; you have finally gotten the mind to quiet so that you can now observe the energy you might not have ever realized is available to you at all times. You are welcomed to enter into a higher place, the "something in between" mentioned in the section on centering. Remember, we are not trying to listen just yet—we are simply joining in on a conversation that our higher consciousness is holding. Allow your inner dialogue to get softer and softer until it is no longer audible at all. Open your third eye (the ajna chakra) in the center of your forehead and begin to listen differently to what is happening around you. Spirit generally does not communicate through words as much as imprints, images, and feelings. When you get those, don't dismiss them or think you are reaching. You are finally entering into the cosmic consciousness of the universe. Trust what you are feeling. Build from that space and create your practice of Divine communication.

Do you hear sounds? Voices? Music? Nothing at all? Notice everything in this space but hold on to nothing. Do not be attached. If you are seeking answers to specific questions, understand that they generally won't come through in this moment. They show themselves after with imprints, instincts, different thoughts, and momentum in your life as you begin looking further into alternate directions for guidance. For now, in this moment, simply allow yourself to elevate. You might get a tingling sensation in various areas, but do not be fixated on what you feel with your body, just notice it and go with it. Ride that wave up.

You don't have to sit for a specific time period every time you attempt to meditate. It can be a couple of minutes or however long you have to give to it. If it doesn't work today, try again tonight in bed or tomorrow. Meditation is a practice. Once you get into any flow of communication with the spirit realm, you will find that meditation will naturally come to be a part of your life. Therefore, don't put too much pressure on yourself to get anywhere fast. It takes a lot of time, discipline, and desire to keep attempting something that can be this intimidating. The subtlety of the communication style is where you need to place your focus. As soon as you start to feel things come through, lock that experience in. Always aim to go back to that space and try to start from there with each practice.

Asking Questions

When we begin a dialogue with the spirit realm, it's common to open with questions in our minds or out loud. Know that any questions you ask will be heard and answered but not necessarily within your desired timeframe. You will have to keep your eyes and ears open and be on the lookout for little hints or messages that may need to be deciphered. When we ask another person a question, we usually get a reply pretty much right away in a voice at the same decibel level as our own. Spirit does not work this way, however. Answers from Spirit arrive in all sorts of ways, and you will begin to develop a personal relationship with your spirit team to learn more intimately the manner in which they communicate with you. For example, it might be in an acquaintance or friend saying something that they had no idea you needed to hear. It could be in a book you randomly pick up, or through impressions or another hint you feel with your instincts. You might just suddenly and very strongly know the answer exactly. Before anything else, try to follow these two rules: (1) Be clear with your questions, and (2) Trust the impressions and information that you receive.

Receiving answers from Spirit is where the four clairs come into play. If clairaudience is your strength, you might receive your response through sounds, a voice, music, and so on. If you are more clairvoyant, then likely you will see mental images show up. If your strengths are more instinct based, then impressions will likely come to you straight through your gut or mind or you will just be able to feel it.

Personally, I receive thoughts and impressions and just know the right thing to do next. Sometimes when I ask the question out loud, from deep inside myself I will suddenly feel a very small thought that guides me to the answer. My answers from my team tend to be audio and gut in unison. I haven't ever differentiated if what was answering was my own voice or spirits. Getting to this level has taken years of honing communication skills. Please don't think that receiving answers via the clairs should come easily or quickly.

Instinct and Intuition

Instinct is something that occurs within yourself, that immediate reaction to certain people, smells, feelings, energies commonly felt in your solar plexus. Your body gives you a signal when something feels good or bad. Instinct kicks in immediately; there is no time to have a dialogue with spirit or anyone else. Recently I attended a talk on energy medicine and quantum physics. The speaker said something that resonated with me and made me think further. He said something to the effect that he trusts his intuition enough that he knows that if he sits with anything long enough, that he will be able to figure it out.

I am beginning to think that the term "intuition" is a simplified way of saying "connecting into a communication track between myself and something greater than myself." It is not something that occurs inside myself by myself. Intuition is something we usually understand within a spiritual context or we wouldn't offer intuitive development training. It's often that the words "instinct" and "intuition" are used interchangeably when in truth they are not exactly alike—even though they both work toward a similar intention.

Conscious Blending

When meditation was presented in my yoga training, it was taught that when a person rises up to the levels of being in communication with Spirit, the ultimate aim is to move higher above those levels where communication is no longer part of the practice. The idea is to raise our vibration into cosmic consciousness where conversation of any kind does not exist. For the purpose of connection and communication with our spirit guides and helpers, however, we are trying to blend into a cosmic consciousness, which is a little different. The idea of this "conscious blending" came to me via Spirit in my own practice, where it was differentiated from "meditation" as it is usually defined. It was explained that in conscious blending, I am lifting my vibration up to the level where I am able to hear the voices that try to guide me in daily life. They said it is easier when we go up to them, rather than the usual asking them to come down to our human level, which is a lower vibration Spirit finds sludgy and dense. When we lift ourselves up to meet them, we begin to integrate this into our daily lives beyond a singular practice time.

Rising to the level of Spirit is what leads us to mindfulness in our thoughts, behaviors, and choices. I am reminded that with every sentence I write here, whomever I meet on the streets, how I speak to my children and family, the foods I choose to eat, and the choices I make every day all have the potential to elevate me into a higher alignment with my highest self. When I choose to live from the higher vibration, I am able to practice conscious blending. Maybe I don't engage in conventional meditation as often as I engage in this blending of myself and spirit for the purpose of checking in and asking for further guidance. Conscious blending could still be considered a conventional form of meditation when thought of as a practice for particular times throughout your process of shifting. One is not better than the other—both are sacred practices.

Clearing ourselves enough to forge a pathway from ourselves to the higher consciousness is not an easy task, but it can be done. And it can be done by you. Trust that and start from that place. Asking the questions you need help with is best done at night just before you go to sleep. Ideally, you are free of mental clutter and the answers can permeate into your body with greater ease. Another way to ask is in the journaling method covered in the divination section. Write your questions and try to answer either in meditation or when you wake up first thing.

Dance, Art, and Music as Therapy to Connect with Spirit

Moving your body through dance, playing music, or creating art is a powerful way to get in tune with not only your passion but also the spirit realm. When we engage in intentional and creative practices such as these, we invite the angels of creativity and abundance to work directly with us. Have you ever noticed that we do not feel the passage of time when we are engaged in a creative activity and it seems like we have entered a dimension beyond our normal world? It's almost like we go somewhere when we get lost in creativity and movements with purpose. This is where our souls come alive and our passions allow us to feel a deeper level of existence. Please make time in your day for some of this to come alive in you, whether it's playing a musical instrument or listening to music that speaks to your soul. If you can, find satsang or a chanting class in your area; both are incredible ways to feel what occurs in the body when it is engaged in a communal singing/prayer practice. Even going to concerts can alter our body's cells in such a way that it makes us healthier and more vibrant because we are doing something that makes us happy.

When it comes to dance for healing, there are many options, whether it's taking a dance class or dancing in your kitchen. Dance is a form of prayer and celebration in many cultures, such as Sufi dancing, the Nia technique (*nia* is Swahili for "movement with purpose"), and Journey Dance with live drumming. There are dance companies such as 5Rhythms that bring spiritual dance to cities specifically for spiritual purposes. I'm fairly certain that wherever you are, there is something—a class, gathering, or event—near you that you might not have known about until you read this and went to search. When you engage in these dance communities, it is a high so much higher than anything synthetic. It is an elevation of the soul.

As for art therapy, it's common in many cities to find classes that are like wine parties where friends come together and take an art class while enjoying wine. There are also channeled art classes that can help you to get into a spiritual trance in order to make your art pieces, although these kinds of classes are more than just music and art for fun. Channeled art classes are usually on a different level, though it is worth your time to find one and give it a try.

When you color, draw, paint, or write with intention—on your own or in a group—it can become a practice that can be the most cathartic form of healing throughout every layer of your body. Creative activity is where the divinity of practice merges with the physical self. The experience is spectacular and liberating; I highly encourage you to find your personal outlet that brings you into connection with the Divine.

Remember: Try not to overthink this stuff. It can be difficult, and will require discipline to keep showing up to figure out how you can get into that sacred rhythm and flow.

Remember: *You can do it.* You do have the gifts to make connections within this beautiful cosmic flow of communication. We all do. Two things to follow are:

1. Be clear with your questions.
2. Trust the impressions and information that you receive.

Conclusion

Healing on a deep physical, emotional, energetic, and spiritual level requires an incredible amount of discipline and determination. It is entirely expected and normal to experience a sense of mourning when we change our lives in a way that requires us to release the patterns that we have built our life around. That said, remember that it was those patterns which brought us here in the first place. You may *want* to change them but wanting and doing are entirely different actions. It is incredibly difficult to make changes that last. It requires you to remove and rebuild parts of yourself and your life, and it has the potential to affect every person currently in your life and especially in your home. The people around you will need to cater to those changes, not the other way around. Stick to your goals, continue to reevaluate how far you have come with every step and every choice, and celebrate your progress. It is extremely important to give yourself praise for each step forward. No one knows how hard each step was to make but you.

You are so much more powerful than you may ever have been taught to believe. You have the strength, discipline, and stamina to make it however far you truly want to go. When you feel like bailing out on making the changes necessary for your health and healing, be sure to ask Spirit for help. Ask for guidance in helping you gain clarity, discipline, and strength to resist the temptations that are around you. Ask to help control your mind and sever the attachments to any actions and behaviors that bring you back to the starting point.

Temptation will always be there, sitting on the sidelines and waiting for you to bail out and turn back, but that's part of life. It's only when we learn to change our dynamics with those temptations that they lose their power over us. That change happens in your inner dialogue and constant check-ins with yourself. If it helps, set up a team around you to keep you accountable, or maybe put a calendar on your wall and mark every day that you stuck to whatever goals and guidelines you put up for yourself. Create a system that will help you make the changes you want and need in order to shift and heal into your best self. Behaviors that cause you strife are so fleeting—simple pleasures within your old routine—it's up to you to find new ways of finding pleasure that stay within the parameters of your new groove in life. If it's food or an attachment to a person or behavior, the rewards become fewer and fewer when you continue to engage in behaviors you know do not serve you. Breaking any addiction cycle is a daunting task, but you can do it.

There is an ever-moving rhythm to life. Every good thing changes, every hard thing changes, and we need to hold on tight to the really good days. We also need to be thankful for the uneventful days in our lives, as those are sacred. Those are going to be some of the days you look back on and realize were among the most special.

In the same way that nothing in the body operates independently, nothing outside of us does either. You are a sacred and valuable part of the Universe—we need you in it! We need you to give to yourself the best chances for elevation and ultimate health and healing in your life. In this exact moment, reach up and grab a "now." Bring it to your chest … and it has already become a "then." Everything flies by if we don't stop to notice the little things. Wherever you are on your healing continuum, keep pressing on. Life is so very precious; we need to treat it with more reverence and respect throughout our days.

Remember to keep checking in and asking yourself who you are, what you want, and what you are willing to do to get it. Practice this on a daily basis and notice how laser focused you become on your path to greatness. I want you to have your very best life! I want you to love yourself and the life you are creating! I want you to know that you deserve the good life and you are allowed to be healthy and happy in it! I want you to do the work required for you to know without a doubt that you earned this healthy and radiant life.

I once read a quote (author unknown) that really motivates me: "Someone once told me the definition of hell; on the last day on earth, the person you could have become will meet the person you became." The sentiment is very powerful, and I've never forgotten it. Every single person born upon this earth has within them a special seed all their own. The goal is to find it and let it blossom into something beautiful and meaningful. We are all gifted in some form or another. We can choose to use those gifts or bury those gifts. Whatever seed that was planted within you deserves the chance to grow into something that makes you feel fully alive. Remember your seed, wake your soul up, and be reminded of who you really are and what you are here to do. (It was never to fritter your life away.)

It is up to you to constantly check in with your spiritual self and notice whether you are in alignment with the greatest outcomes every step of the way. If you're not, reset and start again. It's never too late to begin again as long as you are here and living. Remember where there is breath, there is hope. Keep using your long and soft breaths to propel you into a calmer mind and a clearer path. You can do anything you decide to act on.

You are a unique and special person. You deserve all the wonderful things that this life has to offer. You are powerful beyond measure. No more playing small to your life; we don't have time for that anymore. Your life is precious and it's yours. Let your light shine. Stop being afraid that things won't go well. Trust that when you listen to your inner voice, things will go beyond your original expectations. You are a magical, sparkly member of this universal family, and you matter. You are strong. You are wise. You listen and you follow your instincts. You trust. You are aware. You are beautiful. You are sexy. You are worthy. You are destined to live this life to the fullest. Give yourself permission to do so now.

It is your divine right to live happy, healthy, and free.

So it is, and so it shall be.

Forever and always may this be so.

With all the love in the Universe,

I wish for you Whole Body Healing and Wellness.

Affirm

You are whole.

You are healed.

And You Are Loved.

Appendix
Healing Systems

The following is an overview of the different healing systems mentioned throughout the book. In particular, the bodywork list here contains more details than what appears in the text. These charts were created to make it easier to find informational sources.

Physical Body Systems and Practitioners

Physical Body/ System	Doctor/Specialist
Skeletal/Bones	Orthopedic doctor/surgeon: Diagnosis, and treatment of the musculoskeletal system (bone, ligament, tendons, muscles, and nerves) of the body. Generally for surgery. Osteopath physician: Joints, muscles, and spine. Treat through the bones and body alignment via touch. For bone disorders like osteoporosis, several can treat and diagnose including internists, gynecologists, rheumatologists, endocrinologists, and geriatric doctors. For recovery of a broken bone or replacement such as hip or knee replacement, seek physical therapy.
Nervous system (brain and spine)	Neurologist: Brain and nerve issues. Chiropractors: Spine and nerve issues including many other ailments.

Physical Body/ System	Doctor/Specialist
Muscles	Orthopedic doctor/sports medicine, Orthopedic surgeons or primary care physicians who work with athletes. Rheumatologist: Treats muscles, tendons, joints, bone, osteoarthritis, rheumatoid arthritis. Massage therapists work with muscles as well.
Circulatory system (blood and oxygen)	Cardiologist (heart and vascular disorders), vascular surgeons (training in blood vessels and surgery).
Lymphatic system	Lymphologist or doctor with the Lymphatic Specialist title. Hematologists and oncologists: Work with radiology to acquire diagnostics on the lymphatic system. A lymphocintegram can be ordered through these specialists to determine whether there is an obstruction within the lymph vessels.
Digestive/GI tract	Gastroenterologist: Treat and work with issues such as Crohn's disease, Irritable bowel syndrome, heartburn, acid reflux, digestive issues, and GERD (gastroesophageal reflux disease).
Endocrine system (hormones and gland issues)	Endocrinologist: Diagnoses and treats hormone balances, diabetes, and adrenal and thyroid disorders.
Integumentary system (hair, nails, skin, sweat)	Dermatologist: Treats all things skin-related, as well as hair, nails, and skin cancers. Esthetician: skin-related but nonmedical issues; usually treat the face, neck, head, arms, and shoulders. For sweat issues, specialists include family medicine, primary care, internists, neurologists, and surgeons.
Renal system (urinary, excretory, bladder/kidneys)	Urologist: Works with urine, bladder, kidney issues as well as vasectomy surgery. Nephrologist: Specializes in renal care and function.
Reproductive system (sex organs)	OB-GYN (obstetrics-gynecology): Specialist who can both delivery babies (obstetrics) and address issues of the female reproductive system (gynecology). For men, urologists diagnose and treat issues related to the prostrate, urinary tract, kidney stones.

Physical Body/ System	Doctor/Specialist
Respiratory system (lungs, trachea)	Pulmonologist: Works with the lungs and treat pulmonary disorders such as COPD and pneumonia.
Ear, Nose, and Throat/ Otolaryngology	Ear, Nose, and Throat doctor: Diagnoses and treats disorders of the ears, nose, throat, head, and neck. Auricular therapy assesses and treats the body through points of the ear (also known as ear acupuncture—seek a Chinese medical practitioner trained in auricular therapy).
Eyes	Optometrists and ophthalmologists differ in levels of training and ability to diagnose and treat conditions of the eye and vision. Optometrists check vision and prescribe corrective lenses if needed. Ophthalmologists undertake additional schooling and are licensed to perform surgery. Iridology is an alternative medical practice of examining the iris of the eyes to assess a person's health.
Feet	Podiatrist: Treats issues of the feet and ankles, both surgically and nonsurgically.
Internal Cancer	Oncologist: Identifies and provides a cancer diagnosis; surgery (removal), and radiation (removal and halting of growth) may follow in accordance with a diagnosis.
Autoimmune	Rheumatologist: Treats rheumatic diseases like lupus, scleroderma, and rheumatoid arthritis.
Allergies	Allergists or immunologists: Diagnose and treat allergies; some naturopaths also works with allergies NAET.
Teeth/Mouth	Oral and maxillofacial surgeon: Treat injury, disease, or defects to the hard and soft tissues of the face, jaws, and mouth. Dentist: General issues. Orthodontist: Alignment of the teeth. Endodontist—a dentist with several more years of medical training (less than 3 percent of dentists). They often are able to save diseased teeth, whereas standard dentists cannot: Can perform surgery such as root canals or other issues in the tooth's interior.

Alternative Health/Healing	Specialists/Practitioners
Homeopathic doctor	The practice of medicine that embraces treating the whole person. Plants are used in treatments.
Naturopath (All systems)	Alternative medicine through which disease is treated and prevented through non-pharmaceutical interventions. Diet, massage, exercise, and other modalities often not explored in conventional medicine are employed.
Chiropractic	A chiropractor works with the brain and spinal cord to alleviate physical imbalances by balancing the nervous system. Many chiropractors work with several various fields of alternative medicine beyond physical spinal adjustments.

Massage Therapy and Body Work

Neuromuscular Therapy	Clinical treatment and assessment of the body's soft tissues. Evidence-based and clinic-based techniques help muscles release and restore balance and range of motion.
Trigger Point Therapy	Releases constrictions that alleviate the direct pain as well as the referring pain that occurs in another part of the day.
Rolfing	Created by Dr. Ida Rolf, structural alignment of the spine through deep tissue manipulation.
Structural Integration	Based on the principles of Dr. Ida Rolf, therapeutic intervention is necessary to work with the myofascial system of the body. Usually this requires ten sessions to help realign the spine and body by stretching and guiding fascia as well as using gravity to help balance and align the spine.
Orthopedic Massage	Developed by Whitney Lowe, this clinical work focuses on massage applications as an intervention for soft tissue disorders. Requires specific specialized training. Orthopedic massage incorporates several different practices to help with pain management and recovery from injury.

(MAT) Mysoskeletal Alignment Technique	Created by Erik Dalton, a holistic approach to help relieve neck and back pain through a combination taken from Rolfing, osteopathy, and physical medicine. Includes deep tissue massage techniques as well as assisted stretching to align the spine.
Myofascial Release Therapy	A trained massage therapist or physical therapist works with the body's myofascial tissues. A highly clinical practice, it can be painful.
Oncology Massage	Tailored specifically to the needs of clients dealing with cancer and requires a very specific level of training to perform. Specialists work with all stages of cancer—diagnosis, treatment, and recovery for both terminal and survival scenarios.
Polarity Therapy	Based on the energy principles of attraction, repulsion, and neutrality of energies. Developed by Dr. Randolph Stone, the treatment uses movements to help manipulate body energy to balance body, mind, and spirit.
Reflexology	Also called Zone Therapy. The feet are a body map, so applying pressure to specific points can treat not only the feet or hands but the correlating body organs as well.
Upledger Craniosacral Therapy	Founded by Dr. John E. Upledger, a soft touch, clothes-on therapy that helps release restriction patterns within the fascia, working with the brain and cerebrospinal fluid. It was this therapy that helped my child recover. Treats concussions among other things.
Manual Lymphatic Drainage	Developed by Dr. Emil Vodder, this hands-on work helps move the lymphatic fluid (lymphatic tissues carries waste of the body). Lymphedema is a chronic condition which requires a MLD/CDT (Manual Lymphatic Drainage/Combined Decongestive Therapy) therapist. Look for fully trained therapists.

Lymph Drainage Therapy	Developed by Dr. Bruno Chikly, this therapy is different from manual lymphatic drainage in that it teaches how to palpate the lymph fluid and identify the rhythm and flow of the lymphatics. Both Manual Lymphatic Drainage and Lymph Drainage Therapy require highly specialized training to practice this work.
Lomi Lomi Massage	Hawaiian for "rub rub," this practice involves a connection with the heart, hands, and soul. Developed in Hawaii, it is a whole-body treatment that works up one side of the body at a time. It has sacred elements that go beyond kneading and massage. Its movements are soft and fluid.
Ayurvedic Massage	A five-thousand-year old medical system. Warm oils are used in this treatment specific to your dosha. This type of bodywork is extremely specific to each individual person. Requires a highly trained therapist. Check credentials.
Integrated Manual Massage and Orthopedic Massage	Created by James Waslaski, owner of The Center for Pain, this is a must-try for complicated injuries. Waslaski and his therapist work without causing excess pain for extremely complicated joint, nerve, muscle, and other soft tissue issues.
Pediatric Massage	Created by Tina Allen and her Little Kidz Foundation, addresses many conditions at post-birth, infant, toddler, and child stages.
Infant Massage	Qualified infant massage practitioners are able to teach the parents how to massage their infant. Often used in hospitals in the neonatal care units. This helps to teach parents to bond with the child as well as aid in their weight gain through the methods and movements taught.
Tui Na	Medical massage originating from China. Incorporates hand massage as well as acupressure. Also uses vibration and several techniques to help regulate the body's chi. Commonly offered at acupuncture clinics. Techniques include percussion, pressing, rubbing, waving, or manipulating the body.

Dry Needling	Physical therapists can do this. It works with the muscles and the lactic acid within the muscles and trigger points. Many find great relief in this practice. Excellent for rehabilitation after an injury or surgery.
Acupressure	Stimulating specific acupuncture points with the fingers instead of needles. This is a deep tissue practice that in many cases does not use lotion or oil.
Shiatsu	A Japanese traditional massage style using Chinese Medicine acupuncture points. This style can be perceived as painful and incorporates acupressure moving from one acupressure point to another in a specific sequence.
Ashiatsu	This style of massage requires bars on the ceiling as the therapist will work with their feet to apply deeper pressure to the recipient's body.
Pre/Post Natal Massage	For the expectant mother or after giving birth this specific style works mainly with a woman in side posture and many pillows to support a nurturing body. The therapist is required to have specific training beyond standard massage school.
Hot Stone Therapy	Using hot stones to add into the massage to stimulate and relax sore muscles. This is a calm style of massage people find very tranquil.
Swedish Massage	Swedish massage is what many people think of when they think of massage in general. Lotion or oil is used in sweeping relaxing strokes to help aid in relaxation and muscle release. Five basic techniques are used in a Swedish massage to help invigorate the body and improve circulation.
Deep Tissue	Deep tissue also uses lotion or oil but the pressure is much deeper into the muscles.

Trager Approach	Developed by Dr. Milton Trager, a sixty- to ninety-minute session includes rocking techniques to promote motion in the muscles and joints. No lotion is used in this practice. The client wears a bathing suit or underwear, the room is warm, and the table is well padded. The practitioner works in a meditative state while gently rocking the client's body. They also incorporate "mentastics" (mental exercises) for clients to perform on their own.
Sports Massage	This deep tissue practice is used on athletes, especially pre- and post-workout, race, game, or competition.
Thai Massage	Originating from Thailand, a person receiving will wear full clothing. Treatment includes pulling, stretching, compressing, and gentle rocking and movement.
Thai Yoga Therapy	A passive stretching session with a concentration on yoga asanas and practice.
Watsu	Zen shiatsu performed in the water. This gentle practice helps to stretch a person while gliding in the water in a meditative way. This works to help balance the body's meridians.

Mental and Emotional Practitioners and Therapies

Psychiatrist	Medical doctor who works with mental health/mental illness. They prescribe medication.
Psychologist	Specialist in psychology. They assess, diagnose, and treat psychological stresses through non-medicated treatments. Clinical psychologists often work in hospitals, mental health clinics, or in private practice. A counseling psychologist has a focus on healthier populations who need help with their emotional and mental health.
Psychotherapist	This is a specialty that works with the mental and emotional health without the use of prescription medications.

Regression Therapy	Past-life regression uses hypnosis to help a person remember situations either from early in this life or in previous lives to heal old traumas. See a psychologist or hypnotherapist trained specifically in this treatment method.
Hypnotherapy	Type of alternative medicine in which the mind and deep subconscious are accessed to help a patient address a variety of issues. Regression therapy, behavioral therapy, addictions, phobias, trauma and more can be healed through this practice. Many are psychologists or psychotherapists, but there are others who train in hypnotherapy without that background. Look for a person who makes you feel safe and with whom you resonate.
CBT (Cognitive Behavioral Therapy)	A short-term form of therapy conducted by a psychotherapist. The focus is on present issues related to the way a person thinks and feels and how it affects their immediate behavior. The focus is to change thought patterns to change the response.
ACT (Acceptance and Commitment Therapy)	Uses mindful practice to help treat a certain type of clinical behaviors. A psychologist or psychotherapist can use this treatment.
DBT (Dialectical Behavior Therapy)	Cognitive therapy in single session or group. Evidence-based therapy to help treat borderline personality disorders, self-harming behaviors, and suicidal thoughts or ideation. This helps to change behavior and thought patterns.
EMDR	Eye Movement Desensitization and Reprocessing is a type of psychotherapy where a patient is asked to recall a trauma while at the same time receiving a sensory input bilaterally, such as visual cues side to side or hand tapping.
EFT Tapping	Emotional Freedom Technique can be applied in both the emotional and energy body sections. This is a type of tapping on specific meridian points employing neuro-linguistic programming and energy medicine. You do not have to be a trained therapist to practice EFT; it has its own training.

Practices for Psychosomatic (Mind/Body) Healing

Sophrology	A gentle practice to help bring harmony to the body and temperance to the mind. From *sos-* (harmony) *phren-* (consciosness) *-logos* (science and study). Created by psychiatrist Alfonso Caycedo, it takes various parts from psychiatry, yoga, Buddhist philosophy, Zen meditation, and dynamic relaxation.
Quantum Biofeedback	The particular device used in this healing (called a SCIO) is quite sophisticated—it affects you at the level of your DNA and can tell you anything about whatever your body has come in contact with. It can tell you why you have the emotions that you do, what you are lacking nutritionally, what parts of your body are out of balance, and what you can do to restore them.
The Rosen Method	This works with specific muscles and body movements combined with an emotional awareness to help create a dynamic treatment that helps the body to balance itself. Rosen not only created the bodywork practice of the method working with the muscles and emotions, but she also created a specific movement class set to music where people can engage in relaxing movements in a group setting. A Rosen Method practitioner has studied hundreds of hours through the institute in order to be able to treat according to this method of work.
Feldenkrais Method	This powerful method uses the mind to help relax the body and somatic education to help the brain and body reorganize to higher levels of being. The practice encourages slow motion with mental clarity and intention to help increase flexibility, range of motion, perception of self, and sensitivity to the world within and outside a person. It is a direct link to the perception of what the mind believes that one can do, and then uses guided imagery and intention to help you realize that your body is not nearly as limited as you might have been led to believe.

Energy Medicine and Hands-On Healing Practices

Energy Medicine	Practice Details
Ayurvedic Practitioners	Uses techniques from India to eliminate impurities; reduce stress; fight disease; and treat the whole person through diet, exercise, and wellness practices.
Traditional Chinese Medicine	Uses acupuncture, massage, herbs, exercise, and diet to treat the whole person. Look for a Traditional Chinese Medicine (TCM) practitioner or doctor. This indicates they have studied both acupuncture and herbal medicine.
Shamanic medicine	A Native medicine man or woman from various Native American tribes or bands who works with herbs and the other nature-based or related layers of existence to heal the soul and the body. Shamans work within the realm of spirit.

Hands-On Energy Practices

Reiki	Passed through a hands-on attunement through a direct lineage to Dr. Mikao Usui or Mrs. Takata. Reiki allows the flow of energy through the body. A practitioner opens their body to be a clear vessel through which energy from Spirit may be used. Sometimes used in hospitals to help clear a patient's energetic blocks and to offer healing.
Healing Touch (HT)	Does not require a hands-on attunement. Guides energy for healing. Practitioners use this healing method to guide the energy in a heart-conscious way for physical, emotional, mental, and spiritual health.
Therapeutic Touch (TT)	Does not require a hands-on attunement. Guides energy but does not place hands directly on the body.
Pranic Healing	A no-touch form of healing by using energy and clearing the aura of a person. Works with a person's life force energy to help from within.
Deeksha Blessing	A blessing to help clear karma from this life and past lives.
Seven Rays	Works directly with the Ascended Masters for energy healing. Also a no-touch form of healing.

Bibliography

"All human behavior can be reduced to 'four basic emotions,'" BBC.com, February 3, 2014. https://www.bbc.com/news/uk-scotland-glasgow-west-26019.

"Emotional Health," American Psychological Association. https://www.apa.org/topics /emotion.

Antiglio, Dominique. *The Life Changing Power of Sophrology.* Novato, CA: New World Library, 2018.

Behrendt, Greg, Amiira Ruotola-Behrendt. *It's Called a Breakup Because It's Broken: The Smart Girl's Breakup Buddy.* New York: Broadway Books, 2006.

Bouhdili, Nadia. "How Pulse Diagnosis Works," DC Acupuncture, October 8, 2015. https://www.dc-acupuncture.com/physical-health/how-pulse-diagnosis-works.

Asmelash, Leah, and Brian Ries."Broken heart syndrome and cancer are connected, scientests say." July 18, 2019. https://www.cnn.com/2019/07/18/health/broken-heart -syndrome-cancer-trnd/index.html?fbclid=IwAR1DY_UAhZ5S7iAilKAitzRoVAp _qH-H2ClKmA8X9i2KmfBcZQwVNWGltcs.

Burton, Neal. "What Are Basic Emotions?" *Psychology Today*, June 21, 2019. https://www .psychologytoday.com/us/blog/hide-and-seek/201601/what-are-basic-emotions.

Casey, Shannon. "Essential Oils and Animals: Which Essential Oils Are Toxic to Pets?" Michelson Found Animals. https://www.foundanimals.org/essential-oils-toxic-pets.

Chevalier, Gaetan, Stephen T. Sinatra, James L. Oschman, Karol Sokal, and Pawel Sokal. "Earthing: Health Implications of Reconnecting the Human Body to the Earth's Surface Electrons," *Journal of Environmental and Public Health.* January 12, 2012. DOI: 10.1155/2012/291541.

Cosio, David, Erica H. Lin. "6 Traditional Chinese Medicine Techniques," Practical Pain Management, August 15, 2015. https://www.practicalpainmanagement.com/patient /treatments/alternative/6-traditional-chinese-medicine-techniques.

"Dialectical Behavioral Therapy," *Psychology Today.* https://www.psychologytoday.com/ us/therapy-types/dialectical-behavior-therapy.

Emoto, Masaru Dr. *The Secret Life of Water.* Hillsboro, OR: Beyond Words Publishing, 2005.

"Varieties of Angels and Demons in the Religions of the World," Encyclopedia Britannica, https://www.britannica.com/topic/angel-religion/Varieties-of-angels-and-demons-in -the-religions-of-the-world.

Englander, Jeffrey, David X. Cifu, and Ramon Diaz-Arrastia. "Seizures after Traumatic Brain Injury," *Archives of Physical Medicine and Rehabilitation* 95 (6), June 2014: 1223–1224. https://www.ncbi.nlm.nih.gov/pmc/articles/PMC4516165/.

"Electrons," *Journal of Environmental and Public Health,* January 12, 2012. DOI: 10.1155/2012/291541.

Fried, Nathan. "Lost in Translation: Without New Proteins, Chronic Pain Cannot Take Off." Pain Research Forum. https://www.painresearchforum.org/news/92810-lost-translation-without-new-proteins-chronic-pain-cannot-take.

Galderisi, Silvana, Andreas Heinz, Marianne Kastrup, and Norman Sartorius. "Toward a new definition of mental health" *World Psychiatry,* June 4, 2015. DOI: 10.1002 /wps.20231.

Jackson, Eric. "Sun Tzu's 31 Best Pieces of Leadership Advice" *Forbes,* May 23, 2014. https://www.forbes.com/sites/ericjackson/2014/05/23/sun-tzus-33-best-pieces-of-leadership-advice/#4e1223c95e5e.

Kase, Aaron. "Science Is Proving Some Memories Are Passed Down From Our Ancestors," Reset.me, February 20, 2015. http://reset.me/story/science-proving-memories -passed-ancestors.

Khazan, Olga. "The Second Assault," *The Atlantic,* December 15, 2015. https://www.theatlantic.com/health/archive/2015/12/sexual-abuse-victims-obesity/420186/.

McArdle, William D., Frank I. Katch, and Victor L. Katch. *Sports and Exercise Nutrition,* fourth edition. Philadelphia, PA: Lippincot Williams & Wilkins, 2014.

"5 Types of Mental Illness and Disability," UPMC HealthBeat, May 27, 2015. https://share.upmc.com/2015/05/5-types-of-mental-illness-and-disability/.

Nelson, Eleanor. "Teaching the Nervous System to Forget Chronic Pain," PBS+GPB NOVA NEXT, August 13, 2014. https://www.pbs.org/wgbh/nova/article/chronic-pain/.

Paladino, Tom. "PCR Tests HIV, Herpes–Scalar Light." October 25, 2018. https://www.scalarlight.com/articles/?p=1455.

Pultchik, Robert, Henry Kellerman, editor. *Emotion: Theory, Research, and Experience* volume 1: *Theories of Emotion.* New York: Academic Press, 1980.

ReShel, Azriel. "Scientific Research Finally Proved That Meridians Exist," Lifecoach CODE, January 25, 2018. https://www.lifecoachcode.com/2018/01/25/scientific-research-proved-meridians-exist/.

Samulowitz, Anke, Ida Gremyr, and Gunnel Hensign. "'Brave Men' and 'Emotional Women': A Theory-Guided Literature Review on Gender Bias in Health Care and Gendered Norms towards Patients with Chronic Pain." PubMed Central, February 25, 2018. https://www.ncbi.nlm.nih.gov/pmc/articles/PMC5845507/.

Scheer, Frank. "Circadian Rhythms: How Irregular Sleep Patterns Impact Your Health," Brigham Health Hub: https://brighamhealthhub.org/healthy-living/circadian-rhythms-how-irregular-sleep-patterns-impact-your-health.

Szent-Gyorgyi, Albert. "Energy Psychology," Ephemeral Energy. https://www.ephemeralenergy.com/treatments/energy-psychology/.

Terwee, Caroline B. "Successful treatment of food allergy with Nambudripad's Allergy Elimination Techniques (NAET) in a 3-year old: A case report," September 19, 2008. DOI: 10.1186/1757-1626-1-166.

Weiss, Brain. *Many Lives, Many Masters: The True Story of a Psychiatrist, His Young Patient, and Past-Life Therapy.* New York: Fireside Books, 1988.

Additional Recommended Resources

Emily A. Francis, www.emilyafrancisbook.com. Click on the CD tab for free audio meditations.

Amy B. Scher, *This is How I Save My Life: From California to India, A True Story of Finding Everything When You are Willing to Try Anything.* Gallery Books, 2018.

———. *How to Heal Yourself When No One Else Can.* Llewellyn, 2017.

———. *How to Heal Yourself from Anxiety When No One Else Can.* Llewellyn, 2019.

Stephen Watson, Cultivating HeartSpace Energy (video): Heaven and Earth Reunion Qi Gong: Bit.ly/WholeBodyHealthHeartspaceQigong.

John Upledger, "Helping the Brain Drain: How Craniosacral Therapy Aids ADD/ADHD." https://upledger.ie/latest-news/how-craniosacral-therapy-aids-addadhd-by-john-upledger/.

Index

To Write to the Author

If you wish to contact the author or would like more information about this book, please write to the author in care of Llewellyn Worldwide Ltd. and we will forward your request. Both the author and publisher appreciate hearing from you and learning of your enjoyment of this book and how it has helped you. Llewellyn Worldwide Ltd. cannot guarantee that every letter written to the author can be answered, but all will be forwarded. Please write to:

Emily A. Francis
℅ Llewellyn Worldwide
2143 Wooddale Drive
Woodbury, MN 55125-2989
Please enclose a self-addressed stamped envelope for reply,
or $1.00 to cover costs. If outside the U.S.A., enclose
an international postal reply coupon.

Many of Llewellyn's authors have websites with additional information and resources. For more information, please visit our website at http://www.llewellyn.com.